Many "unexplained" chronic diseases, sucn as Fibromyalgia & Chronic Fatigue Syndrome (FMS/CFS), are in fact very treatable. Our published research showed that 91% of CFS/FMS patients improved—usually markedly—with an integrated treatment approach. In Patricia Stephens's excellent book, she shares her journey to wellness, helping to light a path which others can follow!

—Jacob Teitelbaum, MD, Medical Director of the National Fibromyalgia and Fatigue Centers

The ADD-Fibromyalgia connection has been missed for far too long! Ms. Stephens does an excellent job at making that connection for us and providing her readers with important information in an easily understood format.

—Patricia O. Quinn, MD *Director,*
National Center for Girls and Women
with AD/HD, Washington DC

Patricia was instrumental in helping me feel fantastic. After testing, she was able to select the right supplements which made me feel less anxious and full of energy. Her insight into the thyroid gland and hormones is phenomenal.

—M. Sumner, PhD

REVERSING
CHRONIC DISEASE

REVERSING

CHRONIC DISEASE

A Journey Back to Health

FIBROMYALGIA · AD/HD · HORMONAL IMBALANCE
CHRONIC PAIN · LOW ENERGY · SLEEP PROBLEMS

BY PATRICIA STEPHENS, CNC
FOREWORD BY GLENDA H. DAVIS, MD

TATE PUBLISHING & *Enterprises*

Published by Tate Publishing & Enterprises, LLC
127 E. Trade Center Terrace | Mustang, Oklahoma 73064 USA
1.888.361.9473 | www.tatepublishing.com

Tate Publishing is committed to excellence in the publishing industry. The company reflects the philosophy established by the founders, based on Psalm 68:11,
"The Lord gave the word and great was the company of those who published it."

Book design copyright © 2009 by Tate Publishing, LLC. All rights reserved.
Cover design by Cole Roberts
Interior design by Joey Garrett

Published in the United States of America

ISBN: 978-1-61566-197-8
1. Health & Fitness / Alternative Therapies
2. Health & Fitness / Nutrition
09.12.07

Dedicated to the suffering everywhere.

About the Author

Patricia Stephens, CNC

Patricia Stephens was totally disabled by an "incurable" condition, fibromyalgia, for many years, before finding a medical breakthrough which started her on a path to restored health. In 1998 she launched a website to share her success and show a connection between fibromyalgia and AD/HD—www.addfibro.com (new address is www.reversingchronicdisease.com)—which attracted over a million hits, within the first few years, from around the world.

After regaining her health, Patricia's passion has been to help others reclaim theirs. She became a certified nutritional consultant and has been working in a natural pharmacy for over ten years. She attended seminars on restoring hormonal balance using natural supplements. Over time, Patricia successfully replaced her conventional medications with natural therapies. The lessons she learned from her own journey, research, and working with clients, have inspired the book.

Before becoming ill, Patricia taught Commercial Foods in a technical school for twenty-one years. She has a B.S. degree from the University of Alabama majoring in education. She and her husband, Howard, have been married since 1970. They have two grown sons.

Acknowledgments

Years ago, writing a book was the last thought on my mind. The only way this happened is because special people stepped up to help. Without Donna Meredith, this book would not be in print. Her tireless reading and rereading of the chapters, her patient persistence in teaching me how to write, her encouragement, and her careful attention to detail has made the "unthinkable" possible.

Dr. Glenda Davis's compassion for her patients has made a lasting impression on me. She has taught me so much about AD/HD during the twelve years I have known her. I also have watched her guide many other FMS patients back to health. She is a woman of great faith and integrity.

Others who have made important contributions are Blake Brookerd and Anne Lewis. My husband, Howard, stood by to provide assistance and moral support. I appreciate him letting me compromise family time to get this work ready for printing. He has watched my miracle of restored health unfold.

Table of Contents

Foreword

By Glenda Hawkins Davis, MD

I first met Patricia Stephens in my office when she came for an evaluation for Attention Deficit Disorder (ADD, or AD/HD, Attention Deficit Hyperactivity Disorder). She learned about me from one of my patients whose Fibromyalgia (FMS) pain disappeared while taking Ritalin for AD/HD. I treated ADD/AD/HD for years and saw many kinds of pain respond to stimulants, but I did not know if FMS pain would respond to it as well. To our surprise and delight, it did!

Stimulants can't be legally prescribed for chronic pain syndromes, only for ADD, AD/HD, or narcolepsy (involuntary sleep attacks). But most patients with chronic pain fit the ADD criteria when asked the right questions. Unfortunately, physicians who treat FMS don't usually ask about school history or attention span; and physicians who treat ADD don't usually ask about physical symptoms. So the overlap of the two syndromes is missed.

Patricia did meet criteria for ADD, so we started her on a small dose of Ritalin. Her case was more difficult to fine-tune than most. But she has the tenacity of a bulldog. She would not give up. So we persisted until we found a regimen that worked. As symptoms abated and she felt better, she began doggedly pursuing the answers to her many questions, which eventually led her to write this book, sharing what she has learned in the process.

I am, unfortunately, not comfortably familiar with the natural supplements Patricia has taken, although she has tried hard to educate me over the past several years. But I have watched Patricia educate herself about the supplements and successfully come off her medication, enjoying good health for ten years now without medication. She has a heart for helping others who suffer. As she often states, "I can't just take my miracle and go home."

Some doctors say that FMS patients are looking for an excuse to retire or draw disability. But from what I've seen, FMS patients who get well are thankful to rejoin the work force and enjoy life again. I hope the information in this book will help you find your way back to good health.

Introduction

Twelve years ago, I was completely disabled. Unrelenting back, neck, and jaw pain, low energy, and sleep problems made my life barely worth living. I spent too many hours in doctors' offices finding little improvement for my chronic health problems. I was told my disorder was incurable. Medications supposed to help my symptoms simply were not working, or caused unacceptable side effects. I was miserable.

Restored Health

Today, I am enjoying the blessing of good health. Joy has returned as I can now exercise, work, and travel. Against what seemed like insurmountable odds, I am free to enjoy life again. During the past ten years, I have taken no conventional medications for my supposed condition, and the "incurable" disorder I once had is *gone*.

The Toll of Chronic Health Problems

If you are chronically ill, I understand the level of frustration you are experiencing. I remember how low energy, brain fog, chronic pain, sleep problems, and emotional stress drained my quality of life. The unrelenting pain was an invisible invader that would not let up and that few understood.

As supportive as my husband and children tried to be, they were puzzled because doctors couldn't find anything wrong on tests and offered few effective treatment options. When I tried to hold down a job, coworkers didn't understand why I couldn't function. The greatest bluff of the chronically ill is that most of us look fine on the outside, even though inside we feel we are about to come unglued.

Chronic disease can lead to the death of our goals, dreams, and ambitions. We worry about keeping our jobs, meeting the needs of our families, and paying an ever-growing mound of medical bills. Many of us grasp for any kind of hope.

Hope

The final chapter of our health does not have to end like this. In no way do I want to pretend that I have all the answers for all chronic diseases, but my goal in writing this book is to ask some new questions, perhaps some that have not been addressed in the offices of your physicians. This book also presents treatment choices and new hope for the suffering.

Many Symptoms Overlap in Chronic Health Problems

Even though my diagnosis was fibromyalgia, the principles in this book may help other chronic illnesses. Even within a given diagnosis, there can be a wide array of symptoms. The borders between disorders are often blurred.

My journey to recover from fibromyalgia might very well help others with chronic health problems.

Rewinding the Past

Years ago, when I was given a diagnosis of fibromyalgia and learned that I would have to learn to live with it, inside, I was screaming, "No! There has to be a way to reverse this nightmare."

I knew something had been missed. How could anyone have so many symptoms and the medical community not understand the origins or, in many cases, doubt the existence of FMS symptoms? It occurred to me, if I was going to have restored health, I would have to become my own advocate. I began to research FMS.

Through an unrelenting drive to get well, my health began to dramatically improve. It was not an easy journey. It took years to regain my health because I did not have anyone to lead me. When I would hit the "wall" of defeat, which I did many, many times, I would pray, dig deeper in the books, and keep working. I never allowed defeat to be more than a minor setback. As a result, today, my memory is significantly improved, I have no pain, my energy has returned, my mood is positive, and my joy has returned. It has not happened overnight ... but it has happened.

A Beginning Place

If you are chronically ill and have not found suitable answers, you will need to decide if you want to regain your health enough to move away from mainstream thinking. Be prepared to do your own homework. Become your own advocate. Improvement may come easily, or it may take some work and time to restore balance to the body. The reward will be improved health and a better quality of life.

Thinking Decision: Am I willing to consider treatments that are not a part of mainstream medicine?

The Real Expert

Don't forget that you are the expert of the body you live in. No one is more interested in your health than you are. Stepping up to become proactive can turn the tide of chronic illness. You can position yourself for better health by studying, asking questions, writing down answers, and listening to ideas from patients who are improved. Find a doctor who will become your *partner* and your *teacher*. The word *doctor* comes from the Latin word *doctore*, which means teacher. Becoming a confident, *non-confronting* partner with your doctor, or medical professional, also increases your chances of success.

Mainstream medical approaches may help some with chronic health problems, but for others, they offer only limited success. Hopefully, this book will offer you some new choices, fresh ideas, and hope as you regain your health. Some of these choices may better suit your needs, personality, or financial situation than others.

A Natural Approach

Today, as a recovered patient and certified nutritional consultant, I have learned ways to help those with chronic pain and other chronic symptoms using natural therapies. Natural medicine, in general, is milder than traditional medications, but effective. Generally, supplementation addresses imbalances rather than masking symptoms. However, exploring alternatives can be difficult for some because western medicine has been deeply ingrained in us.

I have seen many chronically ill patients show dramatic improvement by making dietary changes, taking supplements, and addressing hormonal and brain chemical imbalances. I am totally convinced that a natural approach is best. Nutrients, hormones, neurotransmitters, and enzymes have a profound effect on the body. Are we born with a medication deficiency? Of course not! But sometimes it takes medication, or a supplementation, to get the body back on track.

Natural or alternative medicines offer ways to treat and correct root causes of pain or chronic disorders. Correcting hormone and brain-chemical imbalances, ridding the body of health-compromising toxins, and correcting nutrient deficiencies can address core causes of disease.

Thinking Decision: Has your health been affected by a deficiency or imbalance? Would correction of these imbalances help reverse your chronic pain or other symptoms?

Attention Deficit/Hyperactivity Disorder and the Fibromyalgia Connection

Even though I now take only thyroid hormone and bio-identical hormones regularly, eleven years ago I knew nothing about natural medicine. At that time, medications for Attention Deficit Hyperactivity Disorder completely stopped my chronic cycle of pain, as well as reversed my other fibromyalgia symptoms. I have seen this same improvement in many other fibromyalgia patients when they take AD/HD medications.

Antidepressants, which are a mainstay in fibromyalgia treatment, never worked for me. It was the addition of AD/HD medication to a low-dose antidepressant that brought dramatic relief. Newer antidepressants slow serotonin reuptake, which can help a lot of patients. But some of us have other brain chemical imbalances. Some of these imbalances are not being addressed currently.

What is extremely important to remember is AD/HD medications, mainly stimulants, affect two *naturally occurring* brain chemicals: dopamine and norepinephrine. When these brain chemicals are out of balance, the whole body can be affected. When the balance is restored, many bodily functions can be normalized.

I have seen stimulants, when the dosage is correct, and they do not work right unless the dosage is correct, stop long-standing chronic pain the first day they were taken. I cannot forget that.

Too many people live with chronic pain, and standard conventional therapies have failed many times. How well I remember the devastation of chronic pain. We need more tools to treat chronic pain. Chronic pain is expensive, and it takes its toll in countless ways.

Another primary reason I still actively pursue the treatment of AD/HD is the thousands of letters I have received from all over the world on my Web site www.addfibro.com. These letters strongly document a connection between fibromyalgia and AD/HD. Many fibromyalgia patients attest to dramatic improvement in their symptoms after taking AD/HD medications. People have reduced or no pain, better focus and concentration, and improved energy and sleep. Also, this medication is covered under many insurance plans. All AD/HD patients do not have the pain component.

The connection between fibromyalgia and AD/HD is too important to ignore.

Before dismissing this as too strange, remember we have no answers for some very complicated forms of illness. There are too many disease states without a cure not to look carefully at all the literature.

The Value of Choices

So one of the questions that will be raised is, why would a certified nutritional consultant even consider AD/HD medications (psychological stimulants) for fibromyalgia patients, or perhaps other chronically ill patients? The answer is, after working with natural medicine for the past ten years, and after consulting with a large number of fibromyalgia patients, I have seen that naturals can dramatically improve health and well-being. However, this approach sometimes consumes more time and money than patient's are willing to invest. People may get discouraged because so many previous treatment options have failed. A good number will bail out before their chronically-ill bodies have a chance to heal. Some just want a pill. Others cannot afford naturals. Some do not want to do the homework. I am respectful of choices.

Years ago, when my fibromyalgia fog, a symptom rarely mentioned by MDs, was at its worst, navigating through the steps necessary to heal my body with natural therapies would have been extremely difficult. Also, at that time, I did not know any professionals who could guide me through a successful natural regimen. Reducing pain and clearing my brain were top priorities. For me, prescription medication was essentially a "bridge" leading to the next option.

I do believe natural therapies can also provide relief that can show up within a few weeks. If they do not, and you cannot find the right regiment for your body, you might consider using the conventional treatments described in the following chapters, or at least temporarily.

Thinking Decision: Do natural or conventional options seem right for me?

The Source of My Miracle

As I remember the very sick woman who used to occupy my body and think about the vast improvement that I have seen in my health, I give credit where it is due. I have witnessed a miracle. I am not educated enough, or smart enough, to navigate through all these treatment options without divine intervention. I have a strong faith in a loving Lord and Savior, Jesus Christ. In the Bible, he is called "The Great Physician." I have spent more time on my knees than in the books. This is my story of faith, one that I do not take lightly; a story I must share.

Why Did I Feel Compelled to Write This Book?

After working with clients in a natural pharmacy for over ten years with various chronic illnesses and others with fibromyalgia on the Internet, *I find the majority is unaware of the impact that hormonal and brain chemical imbalances have on their health and well-being.* So many are looking for structural abnormalities when, in reality, chemical imbalance can throw off the delicate rhythm that commands healthy bodily functions.

Also, toxins have a powerful effect on our bodies. Many of us suspect their power to harm our health, but many do not know how to tackle the toxic overload that lies within.

Another reason I felt compelled to write this book is large numbers of fibromyalgia, and other chronically ill people, have not found conventional or alternative treatments that really improve their quality of life. I know so many who live daily with almost unbearable pain, low energy, mood problems, and the like.

I feel better than anyone I know with a fibromyalgia diagnosis. In fact I am sure I could not be diagnosed with it today. This book is my way of putting my hand back in to help others.

Finding Professional Help

If you desire to pursue naturals, your first challenge is to find a doctor open to natural therapies. Many doctors will discredit ideas that are not in their journals. If your doctor is close-minded and you are not getting better, seek another physician. Look around. Trained professionals are out there. Do some Internet research.

If you seek a medical professional regarding hormonal or brain chemical imbalance, be highly selective. Become an educated, *nonthreatening* partner. If you are seeking someone to help with hormonal imbalance, you might call a local compounding pharmacist to ask for recommendations.

A Happy Ending after a Long Journey

I have spent years working my way through all of this, and there have been so many obstacles and setbacks. But defeat inspired courage to try again … and again. Nothing kept me from forging ahead to my dream of better health. What I hope to bring to you are lessons I have learned on my journey back to health in order that the road may be shorter for you. I want you to get well. It is also high time that the world, especially our families, know we are not given to weakness, but that we instead possess courage and determination beyond their wildest imaginations.

Restoring Health Can Require Work

As you consider the materials in this book, remember that what I am sharing can take some time and work. Balancing the endocrine system and brain chemicals can happen easily for some, but it requires more work for others. Hopefully, the information in this book will help shorten your journey. Remember, there is no dress rehearsal for life. Go out there and become a partner in order to improve your own health. As you improve, share your story with others. You must because it gives hope, and hope is one of the most powerful medications of all.

Important Disclaimer

This book is written from a recovered patient's perspective. I have learned a great deal on this journey of recovery. Because I am not a trained medical professional, I have included many quotes from trained medical professionals. In no way does this information replace the advice of your physician.

The information included on natural medicine is derived from research, seminars, books, and working with clients for over ten years. All information is provided for educational purposes only and not intended to be used to diagnose, prevent, treat, or cure any disease. Each patient is biologically unique. Supplements as well as drugs can affect each of us differently. Dosing supplements and medications can be extremely important to the success of the treatment program. Find a doctor or a trained professional you trust. Consult with him or her before starting any program or therapy.

Restored Health:
Against All Odds

Living without pain gives life a whole new perspective. Years ago, when I was in the full throes of illness, recovery seemed impossible. Against all odds, my body has healed from a disorder doctors said was incurable. I have seen a miracle, one I hope will inspire you and give you hope.

I was sick for seven years before I got a diagnosis. Those years took me from doctor to doctor, looking for answers inside the mainstream medical system. I *knew* there had to be an answer, one that would release my body from chronic pain, low energy, and other debilitating symptoms. Even though medical tests revealed nothing of significance and many doctors concluded my illness was all in my mind, I knew I was not imagining my symptoms.

The irony is they were right. It *was* in my mind, but not in the way they thought. Balancing my brain chemicals and hormones first brought me out of pain and restored my quality of life. Personal weakness did not cause my illness, as many of my doctors imagined. Actual chemical imbalances in my brain were making my body dance out of step to a rhythm of its own.

Most people think when the body is sick, structural abnormalities are the problem. In reality, enormous problems result from chemical imbalances. We are chemical factories, and chemistry controls everything.

I have worked with large numbers of people age forty and over. One conclusion I've drawn is they are more prone to have chemical imbalance problems than structural problems. Structural problems can be significant, but we often place too much blame on them. In general, the medical community attempts to control our symptoms instead of addressing the chemical imbalances or nutritional deficiencies that are responsible.

Beginning Signs of Chronic Illness

When I turned forty, I experienced sudden-onset symptoms, such as intense neck, back, and jaw pain in the temporomandibular joint (TMJ). After sleeping soundly for my first forty years, I could no longer sleep through the night. Memory lapses, anxiety, irritable bowel syndrome, headaches, low energy, urinary frequency, and low-grade infections followed. Also, my allergies flared to an all-time high, and I developed an irregular heartbeat.

It was an almost overwhelming challenge to care for my family and continue to teach in the midst of the misery. Yet, all the while, I looked fine.

An Elusive Diagnosis

After finally being diagnosed with fibromyalgia, the relief of having a diagnosis was short-lived because the doctor explained that there was no cure and the treatment options were not very effective. I left his office with *no* hope. A trail of tears followed me out the door.

Even at that moment, when the odds were stacked heavily against me, I thought to myself, *There has to be a way to get well.* There was!

Then and Now

Today, my neck and back pain is completely gone. Long gone is the nightly routine of putting heat on my neck and back to ease off to less-than-restful sleep. I now sleep without medication.

The TMJ (Temporomandibular Joint) problems were so significant I ate only soft foods for nearly seven years. In an attempt to help, a well-meaning physical therapist accidentally pulled my jaw joint completely out of joint. I had two surgeries on my jaw joint, one which was unnecessary. On the advice of three doctors, I also had my upper and lower jaws totally restructured in hopes of relieving the pain. Nothing worked.

I later found out that I did not have structural problems but chemical problems. Correcting the chemical imbalances completely stopped the pain. Today, I can eat anything I want with no jaw pain, a source of great joy to me. This reversal of my TMJ symptoms has caused the dentists and doctors who treated me to scratch their heads.

The memory problems that kept me from recalling

lessons I had taught my students for over twenty years have dramatically improved.

Previously, doctors treated my anxiety with benzodiazepines. Working to get off these addictive medications was one of my greatest challenges, but I succeeded.

The irritable bowel syndrome that caused me great distress is basically gone. Headaches that plagued me daily have completely disappeared after balancing my hormones and brain chemicals.

After being a high-energy person for the first forty years of my life, I felt extremely tired. I still had a full schedule, but my energy no longer rose to meet the demands of my life. At one point, I could hardly walk across the room. Today, I have plenty of energy to work all day. I pace myself because I know I have limits. However, at the time of this writing, I am sixty-one and feel well.

Urinary frequency and low-grade infection kept me close to the bathroom, which interfered with my work life. For teachers, bathroom breaks are at a premium. I took antibiotics for about a year, which did not help. Balancing my hormones and brain chemistry completely corrected this problem. The urinary infections and frequency have not recurred since I got well.

Although I didn't have significant allergy problems when I was young, in my forties they became a real problem. I needed allergy shots and medications to control my symptoms. Today, I take no shots or routine medications. If it is allergy season, sometimes I use a natural for allergy control as needed. Generally, my immune system is strong.

Heart-related symptoms were also part of my illness.

I underwent heart catheterization, EKGs, and stress tests. I also wore a heart monitor. Nothing showed up except mitral valve prolapse with irregular heartbeats. After being documented earlier, the prolapse did not show up on a recent test, and the irregular heartbeats disappeared.

The Hurdle of Getting a Diagnosis

One problem in correctly diagnosing chronic disease states is that the symptoms often encompass many parts of the body. Doctors tend to specialize in one area and may fail to put together the bigger picture. It was so frustrating just to decide what to tell my specialist. How well I remember seeing the look in their eyes as I crossed the line of telling those symptoms they did not treat. They also are geared more toward diagnosing structural abnormalities rather than chemical imbalances and toxic overload.

Moving Toward Recovery

My recovery proves that chronically ill patients can get well. I believe what has helped me can also help you. Perhaps you have drawn from the well of mainstream thinking many times, as I have, to retrieve only an empty cup. Hopefully, you are ready for some new ideas. It is time to stop being incarcerated with the costly, invisible bars of ill health.

In the following chapters, I will explain exactly what therapies, both conventional and natural, worked for me and others. Remember, every patient is unique, and any treatment plan should be supervised by a trusted physician or medical professional.

Fibromyalgia: A New Focus

According to the National Fibromyalgia Research Association, fibromyalgia (FMS) affects over six million Americans. Ninety percent of FMS patients are women between the ages of twenty to fifty-five. Many struggled for years before being correctly diagnosed. Pain and fatigue may keep FMS patients from working or performing daily activities. Often the illness continues through a person's lifetime. [1]

Because of the reversal of my own FMS, I believe it does not have to continue through "a person's lifetime."

What Are the Symptoms of Fibromyalgia?

Fibromyalgia is an increasingly recognized illness characterized by widespread musculoskeletal aches, pain and stiffness, soft tissue tenderness, general fatigue and sleep disturbances. The most common sites of pain include neck, back, shoulders, pelvic girdle and hands, but any body part can be involved.[2]

Other common symptoms are fatigue, depression, anxiety, mood changes, facial pain (temporomandibular joint dysfunction), headaches, chest pain, and difficulty concentrating and focusing. Some also have dry eyes, mouth, and skin; painful periods; dizziness; numbness and tingling; and sensitivity to odors, lights, noises, and touch.[3] Many suffer from symptoms of hormonal imbalance. Others have chronic urinary frequency, low-grade bladder infections, and irritable bowel syndrome.

Other Characteristics of FMS

Fibromyalgia symptoms at times are intolerable. Conversely, there are times when symptoms are mild or absent. Flare-ups of low energy and muscle and joint aches are common, especially following physical or emotional stress. Frequently patients report cold or damp weather, poor sleep, fatigue, or overexertion makes their pain worse. [4]

Most of us easily recognize the waxing and waning of symptoms. However, some patients do not have good days. I was one of them. I do not remember a day without pain for the years I was ill with fibromyalgia.

Getting a Diagnosis

A fibromyalgia diagnosis is difficult to obtain because no lab tests positively identify it. Another real frustration is that most, if not all, diagnostic tests come back normal. (For whatever reason, whatever we have is "under the radar screen" of conventional testing.) Usually doctors diagnose FMS after ruling out other look-alike disorders, such as hypothyroidism, anemia, sleep apnea, viral infections, lupus, rheumatoid

Patricia Stephens, C.N.C

arthritis, and multiple sclerosis. Many chronic disorders have overlapping symptoms.

It can take years of visiting doctors to get a diagnosis. One reason is that our symptoms cross the borders of many specialties. The good news is more doctors are becoming aware of FMS and are referring patients to rheumatologists, the specialists who usually make the official diagnosis. Sadly, their treatment plans often do not dramatically improve our quality of life.

The American College of Rheumatology has established general guidelines for FMS. In order to be diagnosed with FMS, you must have experienced widespread aching pain at least three months and have a minimum of eleven out of eighteen specific tender points. These locations are abnormally tender under relatively firm pressure.

Not all doctors agree with these guidelines. Some believe the criteria are too rigid and that you can have fibromyalgia even if you do not have the required number of tender points. Others question how reliable and valid tender points are as a diagnostic tool.

I encourage patients who have not yet been diagnosed, but seem to fit the criteria of fibromyalgia, *not* to pursue an FMS diagnosis, for three reasons:

- Doctors may attribute all future symptoms to FMS, making it hard for us to get unbiased medical treatment.

- Insurance companies generally dislike this diagnosis because it means a lot of expense to them. Some companies can make payment complicated.

- There is no highly successful treatment regimen in the conventional world of medicine to date.

I have seen better treatment options in myself and many others by balancing hormones and neurotransmitters, as well as other therapies mentioned in this book. In the long run, this can save you and the insurance companies a lot of money.

What Causes Fibromyalgia?

Experts have theories about what causes fibromyalgia, but there is insufficient evidence to support any single cause. Some experts think FMS patients have a lower threshold to pain because of increased sensitivity in the brain to pain signals.[5] "Others think the chemicals in the brain (neurotransmitters) are out of balance, or it (FMS) may stem from a lack of deep phase sleep."[6]

Elizabeth Vliet, MD, is the founder and medical director of "Her Place" centers in Tucson, Arizona, and Dallas-Ft. Worth, Texas, which focus on treating women with natural hormone approaches and wellness services. She is also the author of *Screaming to be Heard*, an eye-opening book on the female endocrine system. Dr. Vliet notes the connection between hormones and fibromyalgia:

> Over the years, I have been struck by the fact that almost all of the fibromyalgia patients I see are women, typically over forty, and frequently with a history of hysterectomy or early menopause. Women's pain symptoms typically flared up at certain times of their menstrual cycle and subsided at

other times of their cycle. I thought there might be a connection with changes in estrogen in the pain-regulating centers of the nervous system.

The more I began looking into these connections in evaluating patients, the more I was stunned to find marked degrees of hormonal loss, which clearly could be of clinical significance in addressing the chronic pain problems.[7]

In addition to overlooking the role of female hormones in fibromyalgia, we have also been too slow in looking at some of the chemical messengers (serotonin, dopamine, epinephrine, substance P, and others) in approaching chronic pain as a problem very different from acute pain.[8]

—Vliet, *Screaming to be Heard*

Dr. Vliet's comments validate what I have seen in my own body and in others I have worked with. Because plant-based hormones improved my health so dramatically, I believe hormones are *powerful anti-inflammatory agents,* not to mention the other vast array of benefits they provide.

Jacob Teitelbaum, MD, a board certified internist and leading researcher in the field of chronic fatigue and fibromyalgia, is the Medical Director of the Fibromyalgia and Fatigue Centers and author of *From Fatigue to Fantastic.* (Chronic fatigue syndrome or chronic fatigue immune dysfunction syndrome is considered a "sister" disorder of fibromyalgia and part of the same complex of dysfunction.) In his book *From Fatigue to Fantastic,* he states,

"Fibromyalgia becomes self-perpetuating as soon as sleep is disrupted." He adds, "Infections, nutritional deficiencies can all, individually and in concert, trigger and perpetuate fibromyalgia. Fibromyalgia can also cause the hormonal and immune dysfunctions and, perhaps by leading to malabsorption, (causing) the nutritional deficiencies.[9]

Dr. Teitelbaum also believes males with FMS often have hormonal imbalances. "Low testosterone is a major problem in 70 percent of my male patients with CFIDS/FMS," he said. "It is very important to check the free level of testosterone, which measures the active form of the hormone, instead of the serum (or total) testosterone, which means the inactive form of the hormone." Teitelbaum notes also that inactive (total) testosterone levels are often normal while the active (free) hormone levels are low or barely normal in most male CFIDS/FMS patients. The report should also be broken into ranges for appropriate ages of the patients.[10]

He also explains low hormone levels in women are associated with health issues:

> Low estrogen can cause disordered sleep; low levels of serotonin, dopamine, norepinephrine, and acetylcholine, neurotransmitters that appear to be low in CFIDS/FMS, cyclic panic and palpitations; decreased libido; and other symptoms often seen in CFIDS/FMS. [11]
>
> —Teitelbaum, *From Fatigue to Fantastic*

Dr. Teitelbaum has also seen how hormonal and brain chemical imbalances affect chronic pain, low energy, mood problems, and memory problems associated with CFIDS and FMS. The good news is that

Patricia Stephens, C.N.C

other researchers are bringing similar, exciting, new research to the forefront.

Dr. Teitelbaum has a free patented "Computerized Physician" on his web site at www.Vitality101.com. It is called the short "Online Program." It can analyze your symptoms and even labs (if available) and tailor a treatment protocol to your specific case. His article on treating CFS and Fibromyalgia with the "SHINE" Protocol (Sleep, Hormones, Infections, Nutrition, and Exercise as able) also gives an excellent overview and is available on this website.

Onset of Fibromyalgia

Most I talk with, but not all, remember when their FMS symptoms began. Often it followed the birth of a baby, onset of perimenopause or menopause, flu, or another stressful event.

My fibromyalgia came on with a vengeance almost the day I turned forty. This has puzzled me many times. Why the sudden onset? What happened? There was no new trauma in my life, no extreme stressor that so often accompanies FMS. Perhaps it was a buildup of stresses. I am a typical type-A person who thrives on "juggling many balls" in the air at the same time.

Perhaps a possible cause of the sudden onset of symptoms many experience with FMS is, in part, with falling hormone levels. Perhaps the time in our lives when we generally enjoy our greatest health is when we are young, when our hormone levels are still plentiful and in balance. [However, I do work with some young women who are highly symptomatic. When testing comes back, it is clear that they are also out of balance.] When hormone levels drop below a level that sustains health and well-being, or they become imbalanced for whatever reason, we can become ill. Every individual responds uniquely to these changes in body chemistry.

Conventional Treatments of Fibromyalgia

There are many conventional treatments currently used to treat FMS. Therapies tend to revolve around stress management, exercise, and medications.

According to Web MD, medications frequently used are antidepressants such as amitriptyline (Elavil or Amitril), and nortriptyline (Pamelor or Aventyl) which work by elevating levels of brain neurotransmitters. These drugs are often used because they can decrease pain and increase sleep. However, many patients notice dizziness, drowsiness, dry eyes, dry mouth and constipation with these medications.[12]

Other doctors prescribe SSRI (selective serotonin reuptake inhibitors) antidepressants such as sertraline (Zoloft), and fluoxetine (Prozac), which can ease pain, improve mood, and reduce fatigue. Currently, three medications, pregabalin (Lyrica), duloxetine (Cymbalta) and milnacipran hydrochloride (Savella), have been approved by the U.S. Food and Drug Administration (FDA) specifically for treating fibromyalgia. Lyric is an anti-epileptic medication, and has had many reported side effects. Cymbalta and Savella are both serotonin reuptake inhibitors (SNRI).[13]

The problem with these therapies is that they only address some of our symptoms and often do not correct all underlying imbalances responsible for the FMS symptoms. Some of these drugs are marginally helpful and often provide no real help with pain management.

They can create their own set of side effects and can further compromise our fragile state of health.

Alternative Treatment for Fibromyalgia

Many alternative treatments have been used with great success. In fact, I have seen naturals work better than medications for many people. I will include the ones that I have personally seen provide benefit. Some mix two supplements for increased benefit.

NADH

NADH *(nicotinamide adenine dinucleotide)* is also referred to as coenzyme 1. *It* helps improve dopamine and norepinephrine, which I believe are neurotransmitters out of balance in most CFIDS/FMS patients. I have seen NADH work well to relieve low energy, lessen pain, and improve memory in most patients when the dosage is correct. Most FMS patients start with 5 milligrams once a day in the morning on an empty stomach. In a few days, if they are not better, they go up on the dosage to 10 milligrams a day. Usually, NADH provides benefit rather rapidly when the dosage is correct. Some need an afternoon dosage, but not all. For a few patients, it can take five to six weeks to show benefit. Persistence can be important.

Even though L-tyrosine and NADH both affect dopamine and norepinephrine, potentially someone might do better on one than the other due to individual uniqueness. Some might do better on a conventional medication.

Those sensitive to supplements or medications can often tolerate both in lower dosages. I recommend my sensitive clients start with one- fourth or half the recommended dosage of their supplements, working up as tolerated.

5 HTP

I have also seen 5 HTP improve FMS symptoms. It may work by itself, but some need to add NADH or L-tyrosine to make it more effective. A good starting dose is 50 milligrams of 5 HTP twice a day (last dosage at bedtime). In a few days to a week, if improvements don't occur, clients go up to 100 milligrams twice a day. **Note:** 5 HTP should *not* be taken with conventional antidepressants because it does the same basic work.

SAM-e (S-Adenosyl L-Methionine)

SAM-e is another effective supplement for FMS patients. It supports mood, memory, and liver health. It often effectively stops aches and pains. Mood usually improves within a week, but reduction of aches and pains can take up to five to six weeks. Dosage is important. Most start with 200 milligrams twice a day on an empty stomach. If no improvement is seen, they go up to 400 milligrams twice a day and sometimes higher. As soon as improvements are noted, the dosage can be dropped to a lower maintenance dosage, which helps reduce cost. SAM-e is more expensive than most supplements, but it is usually worth the cost. It is not recommended in patients with manic-depression (bipolar). Some doctors, but not all, use it with conventional antidepressants.

L-Tyrosine

L-tyrosine is an amino acid involved in the production of dopamine and norepinephrine, two important neurotransmitters usually low or out of balance in CFIDS/FMS patients. This supplement can support mood and energy, assist weight loss, and relieve aches and pains. Most clients start with 500 milligrams twice a day on an empty stomach. In a week to ten days, if no improvement is noted, most increase to 1,000 milligrams twice a day. Some even use 1,500 milligrams a day. More is not always better. Dosages can be important on this product.

Magnesium can be very helpful in many FMS and other chronically ill patients.

Other Effective Supplements for Fibromyalgia

Jacob Teitelbaum, MD, in his book, *From Fatigue to Fantastic,* recommends using supplements like white willow bark and boswellia for pain; ginkgo for memory and circulation; L-Tyrosine for energy; lemon balm, L-theanine, hops, Jamaica dogwood, and valerian for sleep and anxiety; and St. John's Wort for depression.[14] He also recommends NADH for fibromyalgia because it "stimulates the production of dopamine, norepinephrine and serotonin, which appear to be low in chronic fatigue immune deficiency syndrome (CFIDS)/fibromyalgia(FMS)."[15] He also finds 5 grams of ribose three times a day for three weeks and then twice a day to be the single most effective treatment for low energy. In his recent study, ribose increased energy an average of 45 percent in twelve days.

There are countless other supplements that help FMS patients. Some are supplements that promote gastrointestinal health, especially digestive enzymes and probiotics (good flora for colon and urinary health). Other supplements which support good immune system functioning are beta glucan, medical mushrooms, and thymus extract. Supplements can also help with inflammation, such as glucosamine sulfate, methylsulfonylmethane (MSM), ginger, and tumeric. Also, Celadrin and serraflazyme can be beneficial because they lower whole body inflammation.

Balancing hormones can improve a vast array of symptoms, including pain.

Lowering the toxins in the body can also improve FMS symptoms. Various supplements can help support detoxification. (See chapters on "Digestive Health" and "Lifestyle Changes That Influence Health.")

Many are interested in eliminating FMS symptoms without the use of drugs. They are willing to spend time, energy, and money working on correcting imbalances and deficiencies in their bodies. They are also willing to clean up their diets.

Remember, some supplements or medications that affect brain chemicals and hormones work better for you than others. Some get better results with medications, but others do well with supplements.

A summary of supplements and medications is included in the back of the book.

Summary

- Fibromyalgia is a chronic pain disorder often accompanied by a variety of other symptoms which vary from patient to patient. Symptoms may also "wax and wane" from day to day, or they may be present daily.

- The vast majority of FMS patients are women, and a growing body of evidence is shedding light on physical problems associated with hormonal imbalance. Ironically, many of these symptoms of hormonal imbalance are those associated with symptoms of FMS.

- In many patients, mainstream medicine offers little that dramatically improves overall quality of life.

- Getting a fibromyalgia diagnosis can cause problems for FMS patients, such as:

  1. From the time of FMS diagnosis, some doctors attribute all our symptoms to FMS.

  2. Insurance companies don't like an FMS diagnosis because it means many claim dollars will be paid out.

  3. There are few effective drugs to treat FMS symptoms inside mainstream medicine.

- There are good, effective treatment options available using alternative therapies such as bio-identical hormones (doctor-prescribed) and over the counter plant-based hormones and supplements like SAM-e, L-tyrosine, and 5 HTP and NADH.

- If your choice is prescription drugs, consider addressing the neurotransmitters that are out of balance, such as dopamine, norepinephrine, and serotonin.

- Low or imbalanced hormone or brain chemicals can be a significant cause of FMS symptoms, as documented in this chapter.

- Toxic overload and nutritional deficiencies can also contribute to the puzzling symptoms of fibromyalgia.

My goal for you is to consider imbalances in brain chemicals and hormones and how they can affect your FMS symptoms, or other chronic symptoms. In correcting these, you can step up and become a partner in unraveling your own medical mystery. Becoming proactive can help you reclaim your health. You can be a part of rewriting a new chapter in your life.

Patricia Stephens, C.N.C

Balancing the Sex Hormones for Optimal Health

Years ago, I felt forced to do my own research regarding hormones because the information mainstream medicine provided did not correspond with what my body was telling me. To find answers, I had to study intensely, attend seminars on hormones, try various hormones personally, and work with many clients. Hopefully, what I have learned will open your eyes to some new choices and shorten your road to hormonal health.

Correcting hormonal deficiencies and imbalances dramatically improved my quality of life. Hormones keep me pain free and improve sleep, memory, mood, energy, and urinary and gastrointestinal health. I know from personal experience that balanced hormones improve overall health and well-being. I have seen similar benefits in those with whom I have consulted.

Hormones Are Powerful Messengers

On my journey to health, I have carefully sought information from clinicians in alternative medicine whom I trust. Along the way, I developed a new respect for the commitment of chiropractic physicians, particularly Dr. Janet Lang. She is an expert in topics far removed from standard chiropractic adjustments, particularly imbalances in the endocrine system.

Dr. Janet Lang has personally recovered from some hormonally-related health problems. She presents informative seminars around the country, mainly to doctors, on restorative endocrinology, or restoring hormonal balance naturally. She passes this information on to other professionals with the intent of helping others. One of the reasons I have such high regard for her is I have seen her protocols work well again and again.

In her seminars, she states, "Hormones are powerful messengers."[16] After observing impressive improvements in myself and clients, I believe she is correct.

The endocrine system manufactures a multitude of hormones, which work together like instruments in a symphony. When one hormone is out of balance, the entire body can be thrown out of step. The nervous system and endocrine (hormone) system control the body. Restoring balance can improve a large array of symptoms.

Uzzi Reiss, MD, an obstetrician/gynecologist and writer states, "For many women, unhealthy aging is primarily a hormonal issue. The day they begin to deteriorate is the day their hormones start declining from a peak level. For some it is earlier, for others later."[17] This quote clearly describes what I and many others experience. Our hormone levels fall to a level that no longer makes us feel healthy, yet we are unaware that our endocrine system imbalance is creating this chaos. We visit specialists hoping to turn off symptoms rather than correcting imbalances responsible for the way we feel.

How well I remember the sudden onset of my own symptoms. After careful reflection, I remember other telltale signs of hormonal imbalance experienced at the time such as menstrual changes, sudden sleep problems, noticeable decline in memory, pain, anxiety, as well as many other subtle changes that are all part of the picture of declining or imbalanced hormones. My problem was that none of my doctors recognized the magnitude of symptoms as being endocrine (hormone) related.

One of the main reasons I felt led to write this book is most of my clients have no concept of the large array of symptoms that can stem from hormonal imbalance. We have been trained to accept the idea of specialty medicine, which treats every body part as a separate entity. In reality, all parts are integrated into a whole, especially concerning chemical or hormonal imbalances.

Safety Concerns

A large percentage of women who hear the word *hormone* probably think *risk* before they think *benefit*. We remember the result of the Women's Health Initiative Study of April 2004 describing the dangers of conventional hormone replacement therapy. Many women abruptly discontinued their hormones and experienced a return of sleep problems, headaches, vaginal dryness, hot flashes, mood disorders, low energy, and a variety of other discomforts. These symptoms can vary in degree from an inconvenience to total incapacitation.

Because of this study, many women distrust the safety of all forms of hormone replacement. It is sad that many women are not informed about bio-identical/ human identical hormones, or over-the-counter, plant-based hormones. In the ten years I have worked with natural hormones, I have found them safe and very effective when the *dosage is correct. There is a vast difference between a synthetic and a natural hormone.*

Any hormone, synthetic or natural, can cause problems when the dosage is too high.

So how do you protect yourself from high hormone levels? The answer is by monitoring your levels. Saliva tests are inexpensive ways to make sure you are in balance. Monitor regularly until you find the right replacement regimen. Feeling well is a usually a good indication you are in balance.

C. W. Randolph, Jr., MD, R. Ph, has written an excellent book, *From Hormone Hell to Hormone Well.* He is a board-certified obstetrician and gynecologist, as well as a registered pharmacist, who has helped thousands of women with hormonal imbalance. He is also the founder of The Natural Hormone Institute of America. In his book, he states that "synthetic hormone compounds have chemical molecules that have been forcibly joined together via laboratory synthesis." These synthetic or conjugated hormones can be patented, thereby giving the pharmaceutical company manufacturer exclusive ownership of both the chemical formula and the revenue the patented product generates for a period of time. Synthetic hormones can lead to health dangers. "Synthetic hormones are not an exact fit for the human body's hormone receptor sites; they are not the right key for the lock," said Dr. Randolph.[18]

Dr. Randolph also explains why bio-identical hormones work differently than the hormones pushed by pharmaceutical companies:

> Because they are molecularly different in structure than the hormones they were designed to replace, synthetic hormones act as a foreign substance within the human body.
>
> As a result, their effects are not consistent with the body's normal biochemistry. The fact that synthetic HRT (hormone replacement therapy) has been found to cause many unpredictable and harmful side effects comes down to a single fact: when it comes to replicating the biochemistry of a human body, *almost* the same molecular structure is not good enough.
>
> In contrast, human-identical hormones have a molecular structure that exactly matches the molecular structure of the hormones produced by the female body. This means that, when human identical hormones enter the bloodstream, they look and perform just like the original hormones they were designed to replicate … They enter the bloodstream, attach to the appropriate receptor locks and safely and effectively reestablish optimum hormonal equilibrium.[19]
>
> —Randolph, *From Hormone Hell to Hormone Well*

When I was using prescription hormones that were not bio-identical, I had a variety of side effects, such as clotting in the legs and heart palpitations. I did not experience these same side effects with the right dosage of bio-identical hormones. Many other women have also experienced side effects with patented prescription hormones.

Hormones are critical to good health. In our youth, when our hormones are in better balance, we generally enjoy our highest quality of life. We have more energy, less weight gain, fewer aches and pains, and better mood, libido, and memory. Balanced hormone levels have never been the problem; but instead, symptoms result when our hormone levels are low, or out of balance. There are excellent ways to monitor these levels to ensure balance.

An Orchestra of Hormones

Often, when the word *hormone* is mentioned, women think about estrogen, and men think about testosterone. The truth is that our endocrine system works like a carefully orchestrated symphony composed of a vast array of hormones. Other critical hormones are progesterone, thyroid, cortisol, DHEA, melatonin, pregnenolone, and growth hormone.

The Role of Hormones

Every cell in the body is influenced by hormones. When a deficiency or imbalance occurs, many symptoms can result, depending on the degree of imbalance and genetic uniqueness.

Patricia Stephens, C.N.C

> When hormonal balance is restored, many symptoms disappear.

Estrogen

Estrogen is a primary hormone for women. When it is low, the deficiency can impact our quality of life. In a premenopausal state, our estrogen cycles and its level is influenced by many factors.

Women can have low estrogen before their periods, after childbirth, and in menopause. The balance of hormones often shifts in women as they approach menopause. This change can begin for some women as early as their mid-thirties. Some see imbalances much earlier. (I believe high stress can be a contributor.)

Symptoms of estrogen deficiency are depression, sleep disturbance, anxiety, panic, difficulty concentrating, mood swings, memory problems, hot flashes, dry eyes, dry skin, vaginal dryness and thinning, decreased sexual response, decreased breast size, osteoporosis, increased risk of heart disease, and headaches. Women may also experience less energy, stamina, and drive.[20]

Christiane Northrup, MD (obstetrician/gynecologist), best selling author of *The Wisdom of Menopause*, states, "Women with estrogen depletion may also experience urinary problems such as recurrent urinary tract infections or even stress urinary incontinence."[21]

In the past, I experienced urinary frequency and chronic, recurring infection that lasted for years. After getting my hormones balanced, these symptoms have not returned. I have also seen this benefit from hormone replacement in other women.

Sandy

Sandy is in her seventies, and has overactive bladder, which is a sudden and often uncontrollable urge to urinate. She had tried many different treatments without success.

After consulting with her, she was surprised when I asked her if she was having any hot flashes, night sweats, mood and sleep problems, or low energy. She said she was having some of these symptoms. I suggested that she try a product that affects estrogen and progesterone. (See Chapter Six) In three days, she called me with such excitement. She said, "It is a miracle! All urinary over activity has stopped! My bladder is functioning normally for the first time in a long time."

Bio-identical or plant-based hormones are an exact replica of what our own bodies make. They can correct a wide array of symptoms throughout the body. Hormones are, indeed, powerful messengers.

Progesterone

Progesterone is another primary hormone for women. The balance or ratio between estrogen and progesterone is critical to a woman's health. "Progesterone only functions correctly when it is in the right proportion with estrogen, its primary partner. Estrogen is necessary to create progesterone receptors, and progesterone regulates estrogen receptors."[22] Hormones must be balanced to achieve optimal health.

In the eyes of conventional medicine, progesterone seems to have merit only in fertility, pregnancy, and protection of the uterus. At the time of this writing, most physicians overlook the benefits of progesterone in postmenopausal patients.

If doctors prescribe progesterone in pre-menopausal women, they often order conjugated progesterone, such as Provera. This form of progesterone has been changed in order to be patented, and it has a history of side effects. These same side effects are not associated with natural progesterone, as long as the *dosage is correct*.

Dr. Randolph lists the benefits of natural progesterone supplementation in deficient patients:

1. protects against breast cancer
2. maintains pregnancy
3. stimulates bone building that can prevent or treat osteoporosis
4. helps calm the body and improve mood
5. prevents water retention
6. assists in balancing blood sugar levels
7. maintains libido
8. helps to normalize sleep
9. corrects headaches
10. protects against uterine cancer
11. improves mental acuity and memory [23]

    —Randolph, *From Hormone Hell to Hormone Well*

Progesterone is an important precursor for cortisol, one of our stress-handling hormones.

I have watched it reverse a multitude of symptoms, including chronic headaches.

For me, progesterone is calming, improves brain clarity, improves sleep, and seems to help stabilize my blood sugar.

As you can see, many health problems are associated with deficiencies of progesterone.

Kim

Kim came in seeking help for her fibromyalgia. Usually, fibromyalgia patients do not look sick, but you could look at her and see that she felt like she was at death's door. In fact, those were her words. She had visited a multitude of doctors and had a lot of medical testing. As usual, testing came back "normal." Last year, she had five hospital stays, and no one could figure out what was going on.

We decided to test her hormones. Her estrogen levels were normal, but she had very low progesterone levels. She also had a high nighttime cortisol. We used a small number of supplements to get started. She began with sublingual (dissolved under the tongue) progesterone called Progon B. She began on day fourteen of her cycle with one at bedtime. After a few days, I suggested that she try one twice a day. She did not see significant changes until she was taking two twice a day from day fourteen to day twenty-seven or day twenty-eight of her cycle. If she went up higher, she had problems. She also started taking 100 milligrams of phosphatidylserine an hour before bed and a B complex. Within a few days, she was much better. She later found that if she took two phosphatidylserine before bed, she felt even better. Her pain was dramatically better within a few weeks. Her energy and mood were noticeably improved.

Unopposed Estrogen

When estrogen is unopposed by progesterone, it wreaks havoc in the body and can actually have a *cancer-promoting effect* at the cellular level, according to Dr. C. W. Randolph. "Progesterone, the 'feel good' hormone, is the first to decline and drops 120 times more rapidly than estrogen."[24] This decline throws off the delicate balance, or the important ratio, between estrogen and progesterone.

When progesterone is low, this can set us up for estrogen dominance, a disorder which is often corrected with progesterone supplementation. Two supplements that often correct estrogen dominance are indole 3 carbinol and chaste tree. Others opt for other forms of progesterone.

Estrogen Dominance

Many women have what is called estrogen dominance. According to Dr. Lang, "Estrogen dominance is a condition in which women can have deficient, normal, or excessive levels of estrogen, but have too little progesterone to balance the estrogen level. Estrogen dominance is common in both cycling and menopausal women."[25]

Estrogen dominance is a serious problem. Dr. Randolph states, "When estrogen was the dominant hormone and progesterone was deficient, the impact on my patients was toxic."[26]

The following symptoms are those Dr. Randolph has observed in his estrogen dominant patients.

Common Symptoms of Estrogen Dominance

- weight gain (waist and hips)
- fibromyalgia
- osteoporosis
- mood swings
- infertility
- hot flashes
- low sex drive
- fibrocystic disease
- insomnia
- fatigue
- fluid retention
- pre-menstrual syndrome (PMS)
- night sweats
- vaginal dryness
- foggy thinking
- memory lapse
- tearful
- heart palpitations
- depression
- bone loss
- sleep disturbances
- aches/pains
- allergies
- sensitivities to chemicals

_____ *Patricia Stephens, C.N.C*

- stress
- cold body temperature
- sugar cravings
- elevated triglycerides
- increased facial and body hair
- hair loss
- acne
- tender breasts
- bleeding changes
- nervous
- irritable
- incontinence
- anxious
- uterine fibroids
- endometriosis
- candida[27]

Dr. Janet Lang also states many symptoms are caused by progesterone deficiency. Saliva tests reveal most, if not all, of her fibromyalgia patients are low in progesterone.[28]

After personally working with women's saliva tests, I marvel at how many are estrogen dominant, or relatively low in progesterone. Perhaps it is because progesterone is the first hormone to fall. Progesterone supplementation, when in correct proportion with estrogen, can correct these deficiency symptoms. The improvements are usually impressive, especially the calming effect when progesterone is restored to normal levels.

Some women respond well to oral progesterone supplementation (micronized). Others get better absorption from sublingual tablets (dissolved under the tongue) gels or creams. An endocrinologist once told me many women do not get good absorption from oral (swallowed) hormones because they can get lost in the liver. Forms other than oral can provide better delivery for many women.

Topical creams and gels can be extremely effective, but they need to be carefully monitored with saliva tests. Some people absorb better than others, and high amounts can build up in the body causing problems such as irritability, sleep problems, and many other assorted problems. Again, creams can be effective but can cause problems when the dosage is too high. Proceed with caution. If you know someone who feels well on them for awhile and then has problems, likely their dosage is high. Hormones delivered in the "free" state, as bio-identical hormones are, are not usually accurate in the standard blood tests most doctors order.

Proper follow up testing can ensure accurate dosing.

There is a very important ratio between estrogen and progesterone. If either hormone is low or out of balance from its partner hormone, adverse symptoms can result. Correcting the imbalance can dramatically improve quality of life.

Testosterone in Women

Even though testosterone is only produced in small amounts in the adrenal glands and ovaries, it can have a significant impact on female health. Testosterone is made from DHEA and progesterone. One of its primary jobs is to build up the body. Some of the benefits of testosterone in women are increased stamina, energy, and sex drive. Testosterone also protects muscles, improves mood, lowers blood pressure, protects breast tissue, promotes bone health, and can decrease cholesterol and body fat. [29]

Testosterone in Men

Hormone replacement therapy is a foreign thought for most men at the time of this writing, but I believe men with chronic health problems should consider having their levels assessed. A pharmacist recently told me testosterone replacement is the fastest growing pharmacology in the country.

In *From Hormone Hell to Hormone Well*, Dr. Randolph says before he puts any man on testosterone replacement therapy, he does a medical exam, records medical and medication history, and does a lab evaluation to assess the level of testosterone. Almost all his male patients for whom he has prescribed human-identical hormone treatment have had a positive response. Some benefits are improved energy, mood, sense of well-being, stamina, sex drive and performance, memory, lean body mass, and sleep. Most see decreased anger, tiredness, nervousness, and decreased fat mass.[30] Testosterone can also provide heart protection.

Some conventional testosterone products have caused problems. I believe the same risk factors do not apply to human-identical testosterone when it is monitored for correct dosage because the body recognizes natural substances differently than chemical substances or altered forms. Dosage is critical. Most men are unaware of human-identical testosterone replacements, which are doctor-prescribed and made by a compounding pharmacist. Monitoring levels while using hormones is very important to ensure safety and success.

Ideal testosterone replacement therapy produces and maintains physiologic blood or saliva concentrations of the hormone and its active metabolites without significant side effects or safety concerns. Dr. Randolph does not recommend testosterone replacement for patients who have or have had prostate or breast cancer.[31]

The onset of andropause (when testosterone is no longer the dominant hormone in men) is usually gradual, and its signs and symptoms are often missed or treated as separate problems without concern for male hormone status.[32]

Men with symptoms of low energy, mood problems, sleep difficulties, aches and pains, and other symptoms associated with aging can benefit from adrenal support, since the adrenals support hormonal production.

Many men do not understand the broad spectrum effect testosterone has in their bodies. When deficiencies are corrected, health can dramatically improve.

Again, careful monitoring of testosterone in men is just as important as monitoring it in women. Taking more of any hormone than our body needs can cause problems. You can feel much better for a while, and then you feel worse as levels climb too high for your physiology. *Problems can surface that are not always easily attributed to hormonal imbalance.* The way to prevent this problem is by careful monitoring.

The Hormone/Brain Connection

Most patients are unaware of the hormonal-brain chemistry connection. Because I am not an expert on brain chemistry, I will provide some research from credible medical experts in the field. If the information is hard to understand, just know that there is a documented connection between low or imbalanced hormones and imbalances in brain chemistry. Brain chemicals and hormones are interactive. Hormones and neurotransmitters form a tight partnership in carrying out many important bodily functions. This partnership affects mood, memory, pain, and energy levels.

One research study shows that estrogen increases the concentration of neurotransmitters such as serotonin, dopamine, and norepinephrine[33] In addition, "estrogen" has been found to stimulate a significant increase in dopamine (D2) receptors in the striatum (part of the brain.)[34] Estrogen also regulates dopaminergic neurons in the basal ganglia.[35] In laymen's terms, estrogen influences dopamine, an important brain chemical that can improve energy and mood. Recent clinical studies confirm that estrogen alone may have modest effects as a treatment for major depression. It is now recognized that an important cause of non-responsiveness to antidepressants in postmenopausal women may be inadequate hormonal replacement therapy.[36] The same receptors in the brain stimulated by estrogen are also stimulated by Selective Serotonin Reuptake Inhibitors (SSRI) antidepressants.[37] Estrogen appears to blunt anxiety symptoms and autonomic reactivity to stress.[38] Simply stated, estrogen helps the brain make more chemicals, such as serotonin and dopamine, and it helps stabilize mood, sleep, and energy.

I experienced complete relief from pain and other symptoms as a result of addressing hormone imbalances, initially balancing brain chemistry, and ridding my body of some of the stored toxins.

Research has shown that blood serotonin levels are decreased in postmenopausal women and that hormone replacement therapy can restore them to premenopausal levels.[39] Many find that hormone replacement is enough, but others continue to need brain chemical support through medication or supplementation. We are all unique.

Another study proposes that whenever brain estrogen levels "fall below the minimum brain estrogen requirement," for whatever reason, and at whatever age, brain dysfunction may result.[40]

Locating a clinician will be included in chapter five.

Summary

- Hormones are powerful messengers capable of reversing chronic symptoms such as pain, poor memory, low energy, as well as many other symptoms that rob our quality of life. There are safe, plant-based products that can provide benefit for women and men. Hormones help create better brain chemical balance, which can also improve mood and well-being.

- When using any hormone, proper monitoring is critical to long-term success. When any hormone is too low or too high, problems can surface. Many of these problems might *not* be associated with high or low hormone levels.

- More detailed information is included on balancing hormones in "How to Test and Restore Balance."

The Role of Adrenal and Thyroid Imbalances

The adrenals are two small triangle-shaped glands that sit on top of the kidneys. Their work is significant, and how well they work determines how well we live.[41]

The adrenal gland is our stress-handling gland. An overabundance of stress, improper diet, not enough rest, or a lack of exercise can all contribute to adrenal fatigue. Because high stress is a way of life for the majority, many could have adrenal fatigue, and we would not necessarily recognize it as abnormal.

According to James L. Wilson, ND, DC, PhD, "People suffering from adrenal fatigue are much more likely to develop a host of other common diseases and syndromes in which fatigue is one of the primary symptoms."[42]

When the adrenal gland is not working optimally, it can have a domino effect on other glands. In fact, according to Jacob Teitelbaum, MD, about two-thirds of chronic fatigue (or fibromyalgia) patients appear to have underactive adrenal glands.[43] As much as 90 percent of our population has some degree of adrenal stress or fatigue.[44] Our "fight or flight" mechanism is designed to be activated on occasion. Instead, we live such hurried lifestyles that our glands do not have a chance to recover.

Conventional Doctors and Adrenal Fatigue

Most conventional medical doctors only recognize the extremes of adrenal dysfunction, which are Addison's disease and Cushing's disease. In general, they do not recognize more *moderate* forms of imbalance, or adrenal fatigue, as possible sources of chronic health problems.

However, many alternative practitioners consider balancing the adrenals as a critical part of treating many chronic health conditions. Doctors realized in the late 1800s and in the early 1900s that medications affecting cortisol, one of the main adrenal hormones, could improve a large number of symptoms. But there was confusion about the use of cortisol in proper dosages. Prescription cortisol in higher dosages caused significant side effects. What was not differentiated between at the time was the difference in prescribing only the amount needed by the body and higher doses that caused problems. [Any hormone that is too high or too low can cause problems.] For more information on this, you can read *Safe Uses of Cortisol*, written by William Jefferies, MD, honorary professor, Division of Endocrinology and Metabolism, at the University of Virginia. Some of his information can be seen on line. Some of his information can be found at http://www.endfatigue.com/health_articles_a-b/Adrenal-the_adrenal_gland.html

Dr. James Wilson, in his book *Adrenal Fatigue*, explains the wide range of diseases affected by hydrocortisone treatment:

> One way to get an overview of the far-reaching extent, variety and depth of the effects of your adrenal hormones is to take a look at the wide range of medical conditions treated with drugs that imitate the actions of the adrenal hormone, cortisol (synthetic corticosteroids like prednisone). The uses of hydrocortisone (a corticosteroid) listed in the *Physician's Desk Reference* will give you the story. They include treatment of diseases and disorders of the joint mucus membranes, the heart, the blood, the respiratory tract and lungs, the gastrointestinal tract, the skin, the eyes, and the nervous system. Hydrocortisone is also used to control swelling and inflammation as well as symptoms of allergies, cancer, viral infection, and immune and autoimmune disorders. However, the effects of your body's own adrenal hormones on your health and bodily functions are even more varied, profound and extensive.[45]
>
> —Wilson, *Adrenal Fatique*

Wilson rightly notes that every system in the body responds to the hormones produced by our adrenal glands.

Functions of the Adrenal Gland

The hormones produced by the adrenal gland control fluid balance, blood sugar balance, inflammatory and anti-inflammatory response, and immune strength and response. They are also our stress-handling glands, dealing with physical, emotional, or mental stressors. In addition, adrenals provide a backup system that produces our steroid hormones when, for whatever reason, ovaries and testicles are not functioning up to par, such as during menopause. They also mobilize us for "flight" or "fight" when trauma surfaces.[46]

Symptoms of Adrenal Fatigue

You will likely not have all of the following symptoms, but if you have a significant number, you should take a closer look at the information on adrenal fatigue.

1. Difficulty getting up in the morning
2. Continued fatigue not relieved by sleep
3. Cravings for salt or salty foods
4. Lack of energy
5. Increased effort to do everyday tasks
6. Decreased sex drive
7. Decreased ability to handle stress
8. Increased time to recover from illness, injury, or trauma
9. Light-headed when standing up quickly
10. Mild depression
11. Less enjoyment or happiness in life
12. Increased PMS
13. Symptoms increase if meals are skipped or inadequate
14. Thoughts are less focused and more fuzzy
15. Memory less accurate
16. Decreased tolerance

Patricia Stephens, C.N.C

17. Feels better after evening meal
18. Decreased productivity.[47]

—Wilson, Adrenal Fatigue

Problems Associated with Imbalances

Weakened adrenal glands set the stage for a host of other conditions to appear and progress, including digestive problems, allergies, chronic fatigue, hypothyroidism, immune system weakness, diabetes, degenerative diseases, and cancer. When adrenal glands function properly, they provide protection against all forms of disease.[48]

Stress and the Adrenal Glands

"Increased stress activates the HPA (hypothalamic/pituitary/adrenal) axis, which in turn activates the ADRENAL GLANDS, triggering stress-related changes in the tissues and organs of the body. When these systems, which evolved to respond to brief, acute stressors (such as a charging predator), are instead persistently challenged by chronic stressors (such as childhood abuse, lack of adequate sleep, or the inability to deal effectively with the fast-paced demands of daily life), they're unable to "rest" and replenish their resources, and ultimately may begin to malfunction in ways that produce illness."[49]

—Lithman, Rodin, Understanding
Women with AD/HD

Supplements Used to Support Adrenal Health

After working with supplements that balance the adrenal system for many years, I can honestly say I have seen dramatic changes in clients, changes that do not line up with conventional thinking on the adrenal gland. Adrenal supplements can stop hot flashes and correct many other symptoms relating to female and male hormonal imbalance. Clients have reported improved energy and a reduction of aches and pains. Other clients have noted improvements in sleep, sex drive, and emotional well-being.

Because adrenal supplements are generally much milder than prescription medications, I have observed significant benefit with very few side effects when starting low and working up slowly.

Dosage is Critical to Success

When using supplements or medications to balance hormones or support adrenal health, remember proper dosage is critical to success. A small change in the dosage can make a big difference.

I will use myself as an example. Through testing, I have established that my adrenals are weak. I am also very sensitive, and it takes a small amount of an adrenal supplement to achieve therapeutic results. If I increase it beyond that, I begin to have noticeable side effects. My sleep is interrupted, mild heart palpitations occur, my nerves feel on edge, and my brain does not function as well. When I *decrease* the dosage, none of those problems occur, and I feel better. However, most people I work with need far more to receive benefit. Dosage varies widely.

When working with adrenal supplements, a good rule is to start low and increase slowly. Proper dosing is critical to success.

DHEA and Cortisol

Two very important hormones made by the adrenal gland are DHEA and cortisol. When these hormones are out of balance, a variety of symptoms can result. Restoring balance can improve quality of life.

DHEA (dehydroepiadrosterone)

DHEA is the most abundant hormone in the body. After being made in the adrenal glands, it makes its way into the cells throughout the body where it is converted into estrogen, testosterone, and other hormones. These hormones regulate fat storage, endocrine function, reproductive function, mineral metabolism, and energy production. DHEA generally declines steadily after the midtwenties.

Several trials have revealed that supplementing with DHEA supports healthy immune cell activity and function.[50] Studies also suggest DHEA can enhance overall well-being. In one randomized placebo-controlled crossover trial, supplementing with DHEA for six months supported healthy physical and psychological outlook (mood) in men and women ages forty to seventy. Another double-blind, randomized, placebo-controlled study shows that DHEA supports healthy male sexual function.[51] Other benefits are increased stamina, vitality, strength, bone density, lower risk of heart disease, increased serotonin levels, improved mental acuity, support for natural sleep patterns, and improved REM [Rapid Eye Movement] sleep (stage of sleep where most dreams are remembered).[52, 53]

I have seen impressive benefits when using DHEA such as, improved memory, more energy, less urinary urgency, and improved mood. Most people need a small dosage *short term*. I recommend a saliva test to determine the level before taking DHEA. Too much DHEA can cause some of the same symptoms as deficiency. *It is all about balance.*

When test results reveal that DHEA is low, 5 to 15 milligrams is all that is generally recommended for a few months. If further testing reveals levels have not been built up, then it can be used longer until levels have been restored.

There was a time earlier in my work when I broke my own rule. However, for me, this is now very rare. I have seen a few who did not feel well on DHEA. However, in others, it can make a significant difference. Just because something is sold over the counter does not mean it is ideal for your body. You do not have to guess. You can test and use it short term when your DHEA levels are low.

Wendy

Wendy, a fibromyalgia patient, tearfully told me that none of her doctors had been able to resolve her intense pain. She had tried a lot of drugs. Nothing seemed to help. She said, "If you cannot help me, I have no where else to turn." The look on her face told me she was desperate and without hope. I gave her samples of some

DHEA and pregnenolone. I rarely put clients on that combination without testing, but it seemed like the right thing to do at the time. She came by in a few days to tell me that all the pain was gone and she was feeling much better. Her smile was something I will not quickly forget. She is still pain-free almost a year later without the use of these two hormones on a daily basis. The improvements she experienced taught me that hormones have the power to reverse chronic pain and disease, sometimes very quickly.

Cortisol

Another hormone made by the adrenal glands is cortisol. Its most important job is to help the body respond to stress. Among its other important tasks, cortisol

- helps maintain blood pressure and cardiovascular function

- helps slow the immune system's inflammatory response

- helps balance the effects of insulin in breaking down sugar for energy

- helps regulate the metabolism of proteins, carbohydrates, and fats

- helps maintain proper arousal and sense of well-being[54]

Symptoms of low cortisol can be a weakened immune system, difficulty sleeping through the night, inflammatory conditions, gastrointestinal problems, and difficulty handling stress.[55] High cortisol can cause some of the same problems, so testing is important.

After working with supplements that affect hormones, I have observed personally, and in others, that your body usually will let you know if your dosage is out of balance. I often adjust my dosages of supplements according to how I am feeling. If it gets complicated, I test. Going up or down a little can usually fix something rather quickly.

Assessing Adrenal Function

The good news is adrenal imbalances can be assessed through saliva tests. For most, specific supplements will improve or correct imbalances.

Most of my clients with significant symptoms of hormonal imbalances have elevated or depressed cortisol. Correcting this imbalance can foster significant improvements. For me, that proves that the saliva tests provide accurate and much needed information to help restore balance, which improves quality of life. I have seen too many strong improvements to doubt the validity of the results. I have heard doctors say they do not believe in saliva tests. They say that because they have not worked with them. I am confident of their effectiveness, when the samples are collected according to directions.

Adrenal Recovery

Adrenal recovery is very possible, but improvements take place over time. Most see improvements inside a few weeks. Some do not see improvements for up to three months. A few see improvements almost immediately.

Lifestyle changes can be critical to the success of the program like reducing stress, finding ways to experience pleasure in life, spending time with people who bring out the best in you, avoiding toxic people as much as possible, pursuing healthy eating habits, and incorporating some exercise over time, especially as you begin to feel better.

It can be important to do more extensive research on adrenal fatigue. The book *Adrenal Fatigue,* written by Dr. Wilson, is an excellent resource providing more detailed information on lifestyle changes, dietary changes, and supplements that can speed recovery. His book provides some impressive research.

Supplements used to support the adrenal gland will be included in "How to Test and Restore Balance."

Thyroid Hormone

Thyroid imbalances can influence mood, energy, and fat metabolism. Hair loss, gastrointestinal health problems, and skin problems can also occur. The thyroid gland also controls body temperature and influences many other organ and bodily functions. Symptoms can vary widely from person to person.

Richard Shames, MD, and Karlee Shames, RN, PhD, are a doctor and nurse team who has treated thyroid problems, including borderline hypothyroidism, for over twenty-five years. They have written, what I believe is, an important book for anyone suffering from thyroid imbalance. In their book *Thyroid Power*, they state, "The thyroid gland is the gas pedal for the thousands of reactions in the body. It influences every organ and cell."[56]

Low thyroid, or borderline hypothyroidism, affects large numbers of people. Many are currently untreated. If another family member has thyroid problems, your chances of having thyroid problems increases.

Why Are Thyroid Disorders Often Overlooked?

Many have no idea they have thyroid problems, and many others are missed through conventional screening. Often, doctors rely solely on TSH levels, when other tests can be helpful to rule it out. Dr. Shames recommends not only TSH, but a T-4 panel, T-3 total, basal temperature test, and Thyroid Peroxidase Antibody to help rule out thyroid disease.[57]

Dr. Shames points out individuals vary in what is normal for them:

> Standard lab tests are unable to identify the millions of borderline low thyroid sufferers. Inadequate testing results in inadequate diagnosis. The thyroid tests used today are just not sensitive enough to identify mild thyroid failure. You could be uncomfortably low in thyroid and still show normal in tests. Individuals differ in what is "normal" for them. [58]
>
> —Shames, *Thyroid Power*

Sometimes people can have thyroid problems when the test comes back "normal."

Other Factors

If you are currently taking thyroid hormone, or suspect low thyroid function after looking at this or other information, know that other factors can influence the availability of thyroid hormone. These are some of the important factors that can make a difference in the performance of your thyroid gland.

1. *Low progesterone*: This is a very common problem, and this deficiency can have a negative impact on thyroid function.

According to John R. Lee, MD, an international authority on natural progesterone replacement, "Women who have estrogen dominance [not enough progesterone to balance estrogen] are often diagnosed with hypothyroidism [low thyroid function] despite normal levels of T3 and T4.[59] When he balanced patients' progesterone, he commonly found they no longer needed thyroid supplements, or at least could decrease the dosage.[60]

Not everyone can stop medications. Some might be able to reduce their dosages under a doctor's supervision.

2. *High levels of estrogen*: Estrogen, in elevated amounts, can block the work of the thyroid gland.

Mary Shoman, a respected authority on thyroid problems, states in her book, *The Thyroid Hormone Breakthrough*, "Thyroid hormone has some chemical similarities to estrogen and progesterone. The various receptor sites for thyroid, found throughout the body, can therefore be blocked—or helped by the presence of estrogen and progesterone."[61]

To me, this is saying normal levels of estrogen and progesterone can support thyroid health. When they are too high or too low, this can impact thyroid health.

3. *Toxins*: Most of us struggle with toxic overload. Many toxins may be tested singularly for their health risk, but we know little about their *collective* effect on the body. They are so prevalent in our world and can take

their toll on us in countless ways, including our thyroid gland. (See *Thyroid Power* for more details.)

4. *Depression*: It is very common in hypothyroid patients. Some studies have shown that over half the people treated by doctors for depression have low thyroid as a cause of their condition.[62]

5. *Adrenal Imbalances*: Low thyroid and low adrenal often can occur together. When one is not seeing strong enough improvements with thyroid medication, after the dosage is regulated, consider treating adrenal imbalances.

Low thyroid can worsen any other illness, and—interestingly enough—the opposite is also true.[63]

Thyroid Medications

For a moderate to severe thyroid imbalance, conventional medications are usually the best option. I have seen those suffering from milder forms helped by over-the-counter supplements as mentioned in the chapter, "How to Test and Restore Balance."

Finding the right dosage of the right medication is critical for improved health and well-being. Many people who could do well on thyroxine (T-4) do not find it very useful in relieving their symptoms simply because they are not taking enough of it. When a patient is not seeing improvements, a *dosage increase will often result in significant benefits*.[64]

Many patients find that medications that affect T-3, like Cytomel, can foster better improvements, especially when combined with thyroxine (T-4). Armour thyroid hormone can work better for some that do not notice improvements with thyroxine. Armour also affects T-4 and T-3. Many people cannot make adequate conver-

Patricia Stephens, C.N.C

sion of T-4 to T-3, which insures the thyroid hormone is delivered to the cell. Some medications work better for some than others.

After having symptoms of hypothyroidism most of my life, I finally got a trial run on Synthroid over ten years ago when my levels were "borderline." I stopped taking it because it was not working. Many years later, I found out it does not work until your dosage is high enough. It is not like a small amount will make a small improvement. As with all hormones, the dosage has to be high enough to work. There is a small therapeutic window where hormones work well. Hormones need to be monitored until your dosage is correct. Too much thyroid hormone can also cause problems.

Recently, my TSH was too high to ignore. My doctor put me on 100 micrograms of Synthroid, which helped a lot.

For me to see maximum improvements from my thyroid medication, I need to have ample amounts of estrogen and progesterone.

It can take a little work to correct thyroid and adrenal imbalances, but the work can bring about restored health. Remember that every hormone is important; and when one is out of balance, it can affect the entire endocrine "orchestra."

Summary
- The adrenal glands are our stress-handling glands. They are also our backup system for hormone production. Another part of their job is to fight inflammation and maintain proper chemical balances for healthy functions of the body.

- If DHEA levels are low, supplementing can improve well-being, mood, immune support, energy, mineral metabolism, and sexual functioning.

- Cortisol slows the inflammatory response, maintains proper energy and well-being, and supports the balance of blood sugar.

- Most of my clients who have symptoms associated with hormonal imbalance also have some degree of adrenal fatigue or exhaustion. Adding adrenal support to hormone-replacement therapy can make a big difference in energy and well-being.

- *Proper dosing of supplements or medications that affect the adrenal gland is critical to success.* I cannot stress this enough. I start my clients with low dosages and work up gradually to avoid problems.

- Because thyroid hormone affects every cell in the body, correcting imbalances can improve quality of life. Strengthening the adrenal gland and improving the estrogen/progesterone ratio can have a positive effect on the thyroid health.

- Balanced thyroids can cause widespread improvements throughout the body.

- Correct dosing of thyroid medication is critical to improved health. Sometimes adding T-3 to thyroxine can foster greater improvements.

- Estrogen and progesterone, out of balance, can have a negative effect on the thyroid.

Patricia Stephens, C.N.C

- When having problems balancing female hormones, work on balancing the adrenal and thyroid glands. Ridding the body of toxins can also help.

How to Test and Restore Balance

Restoring hormonal balance can be very simple and straightforward, or it can take some work. Hopefully, if you have symptoms of hormonal imbalance, you will find some fresh ideas to help you make corrections.

Locating a Clinician

If you suspect hormonal imbalances, the best place to begin is to find a clinician who works with natural hormones. To locate someone in your area, contact one of the labs in the resource section at the end of this chapter, or ask a compounding pharmacist in your area which doctors prescribe bio-identical hormones. The Internet can also be helpful in finding compounding pharmacies and physicians who prescribe bio-identical hormones.

The following are good resources to help you find help.

1. ZRT Lab has a link to help clients find practitioners, www.zrtlab.com

2. Diagnos Techs also can help find a clinician

through their "Provider Directory." www.diag-nostechs.com.

3. Fibromyalgia and Fatigue Centers specialize in bio-identical treatment. www.Fibroandfatigue.com

4. American College for Advancement in Medicine: 1–800–532–3688

5. American Association of Naturopathic Physicians; www.naturopathic.org

6. International College of Integrative Medicine 1–866–464–5226; www.icimed.com

7. Dr. Richard Shames; www.canaryclub.org

Hormonal Testing Options

Currently, many people may not be aware that hormonal imbalances can be assessed using noninvasive saliva tests, which measure "free" hormone levels, meaning hormones active at the cellular level.

Conventional physicians usually assess hormone levels through a blood test which measures "bound" levels of hormones instead of "free" hormone levels. The "bound" level is not always representative of what is actively working in the body. The "free" level is what leaves the bloodstream and enters cells.

From my personal experience, bound levels measured in the blood can be less than accurate. I had my blood levels of estrogen, progesterone, and testosterone measured. All levels were low. Yet when I increased my bio-identical hormone dosages, I felt worse. After learning about saliva tests, I decided to have my levels checked to compare. The saliva tests revealed very high levels. This put me at a crossroad. Which test should I believe? I decided to see if the saliva tests were accurate by stopping my hormones. I felt much better for a few months, until the high levels came down, which indicated that the saliva test was accurate. Since that time, I have relied on saliva tests for me and for my clients.

Why Saliva Tests?

C.W. Randolph, MD provides a more technical description of why free hormone levels are better indicators as to what is going on at the cellular level.

> When our endocrine system manufactures steroid hormones (estrogen, progesterone, and testosterone), they are released into the bloodstream bound to carrier proteins. Only a small fraction of a given amount of steroid hormone breaks loose from the carrier protein in the bloodstream and is free to enter the target tissues. This free or unbound hormone is what we want to measure, since it is active or bioavailable to act on the target tissues such as breast, uterus, brain, and skin.[65]
>
> —Randolph, *From Hormone Hell to Hormone Well*

Saliva tests are less expensive than blood tests, and they can be collected in your own home, making them less stressful to collect. They are mailed directly to the lab.

Dr. Randolph says saliva testing is the most reliable way to measure free, "bioavailable," hormone activity (i.e., the hormones that are actually available to do their job at the cellular level). Because hormones bind to the carrier proteins in blood serum, blood tests do not measure amounts of bioavailable hormone levels.[66]

Deficiencies often show up in saliva long before they show up in blood. Earlier diagnoses shorten the time required to deal with deficiencies.[67]

Eldred B. Taylor, MD (Ob/Gyn) and Ava Bell-Taylor, MD, in their book *Are Your Hormones Making You Sick?*, support the use of saliva tests to assess hormonal imbalances:

> Measuring estrogen and progesterone in the blood reveals how much is in the blood but not how much is accessible to the tissue. Blood measurements reflect the total amount of hormone, but not what is free and accessible.
>
> Saliva glands only allow the free portion of estrogen to enter into the saliva. The portion that is bound to the protein carrier cannot enter. This makes saliva an excellent medium to measure the amount of free hormone available to the breast, uterus, brain, and other tissues that are sensitive to sex hormones.[68]

> —Taylor, Bell-Taylor,
> *Are Your hormone Making You Sick?*

I have seen strong benefits in myself and clients after working with the results from a saliva-testing company called Diagnos Techs. This company was established in 1987 and was the first lab in the United States to implement salivary-based hormone assessment into routine clinical practice.[69] Doctors around the world use Diagnos Techs. I also use and trust ZRT Labs, another high quality lab.

Rita

Rita, a cycling woman in her mid-thirties, came in with very low energy, anxiety/panic attacks, weight gain, breast tenderness, depression, numbness, headaches, food cravings, and brain fog. We tested her adrenal function because she scored high on the checklist for adrenal fatigue. We also checked her thyroid levels because we thought they could be a significant factor. The tests revealed low DHEA levels and imbalances in her cortisol. Her thyroid was normal. We started her on 5 milligrams of DHEA and Drenamin (later described). Within a couple of weeks, her anxiety and panic attacks decreased sharply. We added some Symplex F, which stopped the numbness and improved mental clarity. There was a marker on her test that implied a progesterone deficiency, so we added Progon B, which is a sublingual (dissolved under the tongue for better absorption) progesterone. This seemed to be the missing piece which restored energy and further assisted calmness and focus. I spoke to her two years after her initial visit. She remains well and has stopped or reduced many of her supplements. She continues on Progon B. Occasionally, she takes some Drenamin and Symplex F for maintenance.

Saliva tests provide reliable information regarding hormone levels. They measure the free hormone level which is the hormone that actively works at the cellular level. Another plus—they are less expensive than blood tests.

Forms of Hormones

Hormones can be purchased in many forms. Options are oral (swallowed), sublingual (dissolved under the tongue), patches, topical creams or gels, shots, or pellets. Some forms work better for individual patients than others.

Oral hormones work well for many, but not everyone gets good absorption from them. When something isn't working, it can be helpful to work with the dosage or change to another delivery form for maximum absorbency and improved health.

Complete Hysterectomy

Women who have had a complete hysterectomy often need estrogen, progesterone, and perhaps testosterone replacement for a better sense of well-being and overall health. These hormones work together to provide balance and optimal benefits.

Large numbers of conventional doctors, at the time of this writing, do not recommend progesterone in postmenopausal women. Many alterative practitioners highly value progesterone at any age because it is the calming hormone and helps estrogen to work more effectively. Progesterone also supports adrenal health. Progesterone really makes a big difference for me and most of the other postmenopausal women I have worked with.

Some women who have had a total hysterectomy need something stronger than plant-based products sold over the counter. Prescription human or bio-identical hormones work better for many of these patients. Compounded or bio-identical hormones are prescribed by doctors and prepared by a compounding pharmacist, tailored to a woman's deficiencies. There are a few

Patricia Stephens, C.N.C

exceptions to this rule. Bezwecken is a company that makes bio-identical products that are sold by licensed health care professionals throughout the country. These products can be purchased at their discretion without a prescription. They are very effective, and generally less costly than their compounded counterparts made by hand for each patient. Most of the time, they work extremely well *when the dosage is correct*. This product is my first choice, because it can be easier to balance than bio-identical creams, and less likely to build up. However, a few need something stronger.

Many women using prescription compounded hormones purchase each hormone separately so they can adjust the dosage of each independently. Adjustments are usually necessary initially to ensure success. Too little or too much is a problem. The right dosage usually corrects symptoms.

Bio-identical hormones need to be monitored regularly. Creams and gels can especially build high levels if your dosage is too high. Even though they can be very effective for awhile, when the levels build up too much, problems can result. If your hormone levels are monitored with a saliva test, you will soon learn the proper dosage that will not create high levels that interfere with good health. Once you establish what that dosage is, you probably won't have to monitor as often. Remember, measuring the "free" levels of hormones with saliva testing is a good choice.

Even though I use bio-identical cream hormones occasionally, I got in trouble with them several years ago. I did not understand they can build up and cause problems. The symptoms of deficiency are generally the same symptoms of excess.

I believe current conventional testing can be misleading. Too many of the women I talk to have symptoms of hormonal imbalance even when their hormone levels on conventional testing appear "normal." Saliva tests render a very different picture. I was taught that they measure the "free" level, the same form that bio-identical hormones are delivered in.

Finally, after working with saliva tests, I learned that I needed only a very small amount of my hormones every other day to make me feel well without problems. [Some absorb better than others.] After getting my levels balanced, I test only once a year. Many days, I only use Phyto B by Bezwecken (described below). For me, occasionally, I need to add a little cream to increase its effectiveness. Most of my clients do very well on just the Bezwecken products.

Correcting Imbalances

At the time of this writing, I have been working in a natural pharmacy with plant-based hormones for ten years. I have learned about the following supplements through personal experience, research, and attending seminars that focus on restoring endocrine or hormonal imbalances. Some of the seminars I attended that impressed me most were led by Dr. Janet Lang. I have seen her protocols work well with my clients. Perhaps the greatest lessons have come from listening to the symptoms my clients present and watching improvements after supplementation. I have been very impressed with how well supplements work to restore balance, even when women were highly symptomatic. A few find benefits almost immediately, but most do not see changes for a few weeks. [Adrenals supplements can take up to three months to show improvements.]

Supplements are available to restore balance for women who are still cycling, perimenopausal, or post-menopausal. Many women who have experienced surgical menopause also find benefit with supplements. I will share some that I recommend to my clients, ones I have seen work very well. Keep in mind, individuals respond to different products and dosages. Generally, the first products work, but not always.

Many choices of products are listed below. I usually put my client on *no more than two new products at a time initially, unless it is a vitamin.* We work with the dosages and assess progress. If we then need to add something else, we do. I find working in layers is best. That helps me to assess how certain supplements are working. Problems usually do not occur; but if they do, we can easily remove a supplement that might not be right for the client's individual chemistry.

When recommending supplementation, I always start my clients on a low dosage, which usually does not foster improvements. I then work up slowly to allow the body time to adjust to the product. Starting low also avoids problems for the few that need very small dosages. If the dosage is too high, we can have side effects. What we are looking for is our "therapeutic window," or physiologic level, which is the amount that our bodies need to deliver improvements. Do not forget that correct dosage is "King."

Note: Standard Process and Bezwecken products are sold only to licensed health care professionals. Many chiropractic doctors use Standard Process products. You can contact Standard Process to see who uses their products in your area. Also, your pharmacist can order from both of these companies. They are sold without a prescription. Most of the other products listed below can be purchased over the counter.

A good body detoxification program can help stop many female complaints. I have seen when you improve liver and the gastrointestinal health many hormonally-related symptoms will go away. Consult a reputable health store or knowledge clinician for more information. (See the "Digestive Health" chapter for more details.)

If you have symptoms of imbalance, hopefully you can find a trained professional in your area to work with.

Condition: **Surgical Menopause**

When women are not having problems after surgical meno-pause, they may not need to take hormones or other supple-ments to support the endocrine system. If they are highly symptomatic, including anxiety or other mood problems; I usually add something to support brain chemical balance like 5 HTP or St. John's Wort (These are not to be mixed with conventional antidepressants.) If they still have anxiety, I will add L-theanine or magnesium. Supporting brain chemistry, at least initially, usually fosters faster relief.

Target Goal:	Increase Estrogen and/or Progesterone
Product Option/ Company:	Phyto B/Bezwecken (sublingual-dissolved under tongue). (Testing is recommended because one might be low in just progesterone.) Phyto B improves estrogen and progesterone levels.

Most begin with one twice a day, going up gradually every five days until they use two to four twice a day, or the lowest dosage that provides benefit. Dosage matters and can vary among women. Starting low and working up is best because any hormone that is too high can cause problems. Some feel well on very small amounts.

Progon B/Bezwecken: (sublingual progesterone). Some women who have had a hysterectomy have enough estrogen, but not enough progesterone. Saliva testing will reveal deficiencies. One to four twice a day. I always start one twice a day and go up slowly after a few days.

Tribulus/Standard Process:
Half to one two to three times
a day. Tribulus also supports production of our steroid hormones,
adrenal gland health, vaginal
moisture, and libido.

Target Goal:

Support Pituitary, Thyroid,
Adrenals, and Ovaries

Product Option/
Company

Symplex F/Standard Process:
I start clients on one twice a
day and go up to two twice
a day, if needed. This product is often used for only a
few months. Sometimes, it
is used longer. (If women
have no ovaries, this product
can still be effective.) Most
of the ladies I recommend
Symplex F to notice increased
energy, better mood, as well as
many other improvements.

Target Goal:

Support the Adrenal Gland.
Dosage is critical to success on
all adrenal products. General
Rule: I start low and work up
slowly. Too much can make you
feel off. I use only one of the
first four products listed below.
The following products support adrenal health and usually

_____ *Patricia Stephens, C.N.C*

provide noticeable improvements in many symptoms.

I use these products sometimes without testing when clients tell me they have low energy.

Product Option/ Company:

Drenamin/Standard Process: I start clients on one in the morning only. If they see no change in two days, we usually increase to one twice a day for a couple of days. General dosage, which varies widely, is one to three, three times a day. Rule: Start low and work up slowly.
Adapt/InterPlexus: Most start with one the first day in the morning. Some use one or two in the morning and some take one midafternoon.
Adrenasense/Natural Factors: One to four a day in divided dosages
Stress Support Multi/ New Chapter: Three a day are recommended.

I put almost all my clients with adrenal imbalances on B Complex and Vitamin C. Both of these vitamins support adrenal health.

Cataplex B/ Standard Process: It is a whole-foods B

complex. Most take one to two twice a day with food. (OR)
B Complex: Various companies suggest appropriate dosages.
Vitamin C with Bioflavoids: one to 2,000 milligrams a day.

If adrenal hormones are tested, and cortisol is depressed or low, I recommend one of the following to my clients for at least three to six months:

Licorice (high grade)/Standard Process/MediHerb: Most use ¼ to 1 teaspoon in the morning. Some take it also at noon. Not recommended in patients with high blood pressure. (I have seen good results with this product personally.) I use a basic adrenal support product in addition to licorice. Dosage matters.
(Or)
Rehmannia/Standard Process/MediHerb: It can be used in patients with *high blood pressure.* Most use ½ to 1 teaspoon one to three times daily. Dosage matters.

Adrenal, Desiccated/Standard Process: I use this product one to three months only, with other adrenal support.
Isocort/Bezwecken will also

assist to balance cortisol. I start with ½ once a day. Most need to go up to 1–2 in the morning and one later in the day. I rarely recommend this product for more than two months. The reason is some clinicians theorize that this can make the adrenals lazy, if used longer. I always use this with other adrenal support.

When cortisol is elevated, I recommend to my clients:

Phosphatidylserine: Most use 100 to 200 milligrams thirty minutes before bed. Some use one in the morning, if they have elevated cortisol upon wakening. Working with the time and dosage amount can be important. Serophos/ InterPlexus is a good product at a reasonable cost. Other supplements work well for high cortisol such as Holy Basil, Magnolia, and Ashwaganda. Drenamin also assists in adrenal balance.

Target Goal:	Improve Testosterone
Product Option/ Company:	DHEA: 5 to 10 milligrams a day/various companies (recom-

mended to use when tests show low levels)

Orchex/Standard Process: Most use one to two three times daily.

Maca/various companies as directed

Ginseng/various companies as directed

Tribulus Standard Process/ MediHerb: Most use one, two to three times daily.

If you are still symptomatic after balancing female and adrenal hormones, have your thyroid gland carefully tested. Make sure you are not borderline.

Condition: **Nonsurgical Menopause**

If anxiety and mood problems are present, I usually use supplements for brain chemical support such as 5 HTP or St. John's Wort (These are not to be mixed with conventional antidepressants.). If anxiety is still present, I add L-theanine or magnesium.

Target Goal: Increase Estrogen and Progesterone

Product Option/   Phyto B/Bezwecken (dose as
Company: previously directed) (Testing is recommended.)
                     (or)

Target Goal: Increase Progesterone

Product Option/ Company:	Progon B/Bezwecken (dose as previously directed) (Testing is recommended) (or)
Target Goal:	Products without hormones to decrease menopausal symptoms
Product Option/ Company:	Menosense/Natural Factors: One to four a day.
	Indolplex/Integrative Therapeutics One a day with food Estrotone/New Chapter: One twice a day.
Target Goal:	Balance Testosterone
Product Option/ Company:	DHEA: Most use 5 to 10 milligrams daily/various compa- nies (Testing is recommended.) Orchex/Standard Process: Most use one to two, three times daily. Tribulus/Standard Process: Most use one two to three times daily. Ginseng/Various companies state their dosages. Maca/Various companies state their dosages.
Target Goal:	Adrenal Support

[I often add adrenal support because it usually increases

energy, improves sleep, emotional wellbeing, and libido in some.]

Product Option/   Drenamin/Standard Process
Company

                         Adapt/Interplex
                         Adrenasense/Natural Factors
                         Multi Stress Support/New
                         Chapter or Adrenasense/
                         Natural Factors.

Condition: **Perimenopause (still cycling)**

Perimenopause can span many years before menopause where hormone levels are beginning to shift or decline. Correcting imbalances can improve symptoms. Some clinicians note that symptoms can occur between five and fifteen years before menopause.

If anxiety and mood problems are present, I usually use supplements for brain chemical support such as 5 HTP or St. John's Wort (These are not to be mixed with conventional antidepressants.) If anxiety is still present, I add L-theanine or magnesium. This usually provides fast relief.

Target Goal: Improve Progesterone/
                        Estrogen Ratio

                        (Generally, I choose one of the
                        following.)
Product Option/   Estrosense/Natural Factors:
Company: Most take one to four daily.
                        Indolplex/Integrative

Therapeutics: Most use one or two daily.

Ovex/Standard Process Most use one to three two to three times daily.

Chastetree/Standard Process: Most use one a day.

I often combined Ovex and Chastetree)

Progon B/Bezwecken (bio-identical progesterone): For women who are still cycling, it is used the last two weeks of their cycle. It is discontinued the day the menstrual cycle begins. I find the best way is to start slowly and build the dosage. Most start with one twice a day in the morning and evening. In four to five days, if no improvements are noted, they are told to take two in the morning and two in the evening, adjusting until they feel better. Dosage matters. Most of my ladies end up taking two twice day on day fourteen through twenty-six to twenty-eight. Some need three to four twice a day. Too much can cause side effects. When they feel "off," I tell them to reduce the dosage.

Estrotone/New Chapter: Most use one to two twice daily.

Target Goal:	Improve Adrenal Health
	(I choose one of the following.)
Product Option/ Company:	Drenamin/Standard Process: Most start with one a day with breakfast. They go up until improvement is noted. Many take one to three, three times a day. Adapt/Interplexus: Most begin with one in the morning the first day to monitor the effect. Most take one to two in the morning, and some take one midafternoon. Eleuthero (Siberian Ginseng)/ Standard Process: Most use one to three daily. Other brands as directed. Adrenasense/Natural Factors: Most start with one to two daily, going up as needed. Range is one to four daily in divided dosages. B Complex and Vitamin C

DHEA supplementation should be used only when testing shows deficiency. Then it should be carefully monitored.

Dosage matters on all hormones. High hormone levels can cause the same symptoms as deficiency. That is why I generally start low and work up the dosage.

Condition: **Premenstrual Syndrome (PMS)**

Multiple factors can contribute to PMS. Generally, it is deficiencies and imbalances in the following. Most I work with seem to have imbalances in the estrogen/progesterone ratio.

Target Goal:	Improve Progesterone/Estrogen ratio
Product Option/	Indolplex/Integrative Therapeutics:
Company:	(Contains no hormones.)Most take one once or twice daily. Ovex/Standard Process: Most use one to three twice daily. Chastetree (Vitex)/ Standard Process: Most use one twice daily. Estrosense/Natural Factors: one to four daily in divided dosages. Progon B- (as directed above.) Monitor levels
Target Goal:	Improve Magnesium Level [Magnesium helps calm the body.]
Product Option/ Company:	Natural Calm/Natural Vitality Most start with one teaspoon at bed. Magnesium Citrate- 250-500 milligrams daily Too much magnesium can cause loose bowel. The correct dosage will not.

Target Goal:	Balance Serotonin and Other Neurotransmitters
Product Option/ Company:	5 HTP, SAM-e, St. John's Wort (See chapter 8)
Target Goal: Product Option/ Company:	Balance Dopamine L-tyrosine or NADH (See chapter 7)
Target Goal:	Balance Thyroid Level
Product Option/ Company:	Metabolic Advantage/Enzymatic Therapy: Most use one to six daily in divided dosages. Thyrophin PMG /Standard Process: Most start with one or two daily and work up until they see improvements. Many clinicians use much more, like five to eight a day. Do this with your doctor's permission. Iodomere/Standard Process: Most start with ¼ a day for a few days. In one week, go to ½ a day. If no problems occur, some increase faster every few days to one or two a day. Some clinicians recommend larger dosages of iodine. Kelp: (highly individualized dosages) Coconut oil: Start with ½ teaspoon twice daily. Go up every

three to four days until you reach about three tablespoons a day. Also assists in removing toxins. (Too much too soon can make you feel bad temporarily.)

Target Goal:	Supplement with B Vitamins
Product Option/ Company:	B Vitamins, particularly B 6, has been helpful in any endocrine imbalance. Take as directed. B Complex contains it, but many benefit with additional B 6.
Target Goal:	Balance Estrogen Levels
Product Option/ Company:	Estrotone/New Chapter: Most use one or two twice daily. Indolplex/Integrative Therapeutics Most take one or two daily in divided dosages. Can help improve vaginal moisture.

Condition: **Hormonally Driven Cancer Patients**

All of the products mentioned contain *no* hormones. Some see benefits in one to three months after beginning supplementation.

Target Goal:	Relieve Symptoms of Hormonal Imbalance
Product Option/ Company:	Indolplex/Integrative Therapeutics: Most take one to two daily with food.

Indolplex is made from cruciferous vegetables.

Estrosense/Natural Factors: Most take one or two twice a day with food. (made from cruciferous vegetables and plant detoxifiers)

Brevail/Barleans: (made from flax lignans) Most use one daily.

B Complex: One daily.

Antioxidants: A variety of antioxidants, like acai berry, can be helpful when the dosage is high enough.

Total body detoxification (see your health food stores.)

Condition: **Low Thyroid**

When thyroid hormone is significantly low, conventional prescriptions are in order. Supplements rarely work well when significant deficiencies exist. Supplements can help those who have mild deficiencies.

Target Goal: Supporting the Thyroid Gland

Product Option/   Metabolic Advantage/
Company: Enzymatic Therapy: Most use one to two up to three times a day. Some use one or two daily.
Coconut oil (directions under PMS)
Kelp: Take as directed.
Iodine: Take as directed by your health care professional

Selenium: Most take 200 micrograms once daily.
Forskolin: Most take as directed on product.
Good multivitamin

Many factors can influence proper functioning of the thyroid gland. Low progesterone, adrenal gland imbalances, mineral deficiencies, and toxic elements can all adversely affect thyroid health.

Libido

The results from a study printed in the February 1999 Journal of the American Medical Association state that about 43 percent of women suffer from chronic sexual dysfunction.[70]

There are ways to boost libido. Often, balancing estrogen, progesterone, and testosterone will improve libido. When it doesn't, improving adrenal health and thyroid health can make a big difference.

Sexual problems are complicated, and many other factors can contribute. Depression can also be a contributing cause.

Other supplements that can be helpful for low libido are ITI Woman/Integrative Therapeutics, Sex Essentials/Natural Factors, L-Arginine, Ginseng, Zinc, Maca, Ashwaganda, NADH, and ginkgo. Many clinicians use ginkgo with conventional antidepressants when libido is low.

Male Hormonal Imbalances

Men are finally realizing that many complaints can be

related to endocrine imbalance. I see a steady stream of them interested in enhancing low libido, low energy, and brain performance. Some are interested in testing, and the test I would recommend is the male panel from Diagnos Techs. Also, ZRT Labs has a good panel of tests for men. I would also recommend looking at adrenal function, since the adrenal gland is the stress-handling gland, and most men live under continual pressure.

Many men feel much better with ginseng. Some brands of ginseng, like Eleuthero, do not usually cause elevations in blood pressure, but others like Panex Ginseng can elevate blood pressure in some individuals. A good grade of Tribulus can also help many men feel better. Standard Process makes an excellent product for men called Symplex M. It supports male endocrine glands and can provide improved energy and mood. I have also seen these products support weight loss.

Hormones 101

Even when you are deficient in a hormone, sometimes you have to begin to increase levels slowly for your body to get used to it. Not everyone has to adjust slowly, but others do. We are all unique. Starting low and working up is important because some women only need small doses of hormones. Problems surface when the dosage is too high, which leads women and men to think they cannot tolerate a particular hormone, when in reality, the dosage was simply too high for them.

I have experienced greater success in myself and clients when I start low and work up slowly. Even though it may take a little longer, this method usually avoids problems and improves overall results.

Summary

- It takes time and effort to balance the endocrine system, but the work pays handsome dividends.

- Generally, a balanced endocrine system results in a better sense of well-being, improved energy, mood, memory, sleep, and libido.

- Many other chronic health concerns should also improve, such as less or no pain, including headaches and back, neck, and arthritic pain. Hormonal imbalance can also affect heart health and blood sugar imbalances.

- Hormone benefits are far reaching and vary widely among individuals.

- Currently, conventional medicine does not generally link health problems to endocrine imbalances. This needs to change. Even though the study of the endocrine system is still basically a pioneer field, much information is coming forth to document widespread benefits of hormone replacement.

- Dosages of all hormones are very important. Too much of any hormone can cause the same symptoms as deficiency and shut down the receptor sites.[71] What works is the amount your body needs. The right amount will correct the symptoms of imbalance. How you feel is a good guide. Also, testing helps eliminate guesswork.

- Some forms of hormones work better for individual patients than others. Many patients do not absorb oral hormones well. They are metabolized in the liver and converted to other hormones. Sublingual, pellets, shots, or hormones applied to the skin work better for some people than oral (by mouth) hormones. Topical hormones in cream or gel form must be closely monitored by saliva tests because they can build up in the fat cells of the body.[72]

- There are safe and effective options used by large numbers of patients throughout the country.

Perhaps you will become part of a growing number who seek to balance hormones in order to enjoy a higher quality of life. Remember *balance* is the key word. When hormones are in balance, they exert a powerful influence on the body and improve a vast array of symptoms.

Resources

Quality saliva assays

Diagnos Tech	www.diagnostechs.com
ZRT Labratories	www.salivatest.com

Bio-identical hormones

Bezwecken Products	www.bezwecken.com

Quality natural supplements

PhytoPharmica	www.phytopharmica.com
Standard Process	www.standardprocess.com
Natural Factors	www.naturalfactors.com
Barleans	www.barleans.com
New Chapter	www.new-chapter.com
InterPlexus	www.interplexus.com
Integrative Therapeutics	www.intregrativetherapeutics.com

The Complexities of Attention Deficit/ Hyperactivity Disorder

Perhaps connecting attention deficit/hyperactivity disorder (AD/HD) to chronic health concerns might be a big stretch for many of you. I am including this chapter because I believe the information provides choices for readers. It also provided great freedom for me emotionally years ago when I realized that I fit the AD/HD criteria. It finally put a name to something I had wrestled with all my life. Coming face-to-face with this has really set me free and let me off the hook from further unrealistic expectations. This has not given me a license to stop working hard. I now move toward my strengths and am more understanding of my areas of weakness.

Most of my life I told myself, "If I would just try harder, I could fit the mold." This created great stress. I finally learned that it is not about trying harder. After years of trying to fit a "round peg into a square hole," I am now able to accept and embrace my uniqueness.

My strengths and weaknesses are part of the original design. Finally, I understand and like myself for the first time in my life. Perhaps this information will be used to provide this same freedom for others.

> If you have AD/HD, stop thinking of yourself as defective.

Another reason for this chapter is that, after I was treated for AD/HD, I had complete remission of my pain and other symptoms associated with fibromyalgia. I not only saw this benefit in myself, but in many other adults.

Even though I successfully used stimulant medications for a few years with none of the scary side effects that some of us have been told about in the media, I hungered to find something natural. I also experienced no withdrawal or any other problems from stopping stimulant medications. Because they served me so well for a season in my life and I saw others dramatically benefit, I still believe stimulant medications have their place.

So what magically happened that I no longer needed the medications? The answer came by balancing my brain chemistry, hormones, and working to rid my body of toxins. Currently, I now take only things that boost my thyroid, adrenals, and female hormones. For me, this has filled in the brain chemistry gap.

Discovering the AD/HD and FMS Connection
One day, while filling in for the fibromyalgia support group caller to inform members of the next meeting, I learned a powerful, life-altering lesson. After going

down the list and listening to each caller tell me how bad she was feeling, it was hard to make the last call. To my surprise, the last FMS member, Sara, was feeling "fine." "Fine?" I asked. "What have you done and where have you been?" Her answer would change my life.

Sara

Sara, a fibromyalgia patient, told me about a doctor who carefully screened her for Attention Deficit/Hyperactivity Disorder. After being diagnosed with AD/HD, her doctor put her on 5 milligrams of (Brand name) Ritalin once a day for three days. If no better on day four, she was to take 10 milligrams of Ritalin. She was no better for the first three days. On day four, when she increased her dosage, every pain in her body went away. She had energy for the first time in a long time, which was accompanied by an impressive mood lift.

What Sara did not know is that stimulants, which are used to treat AD/HD and narcolepsy, affect chemicals that naturally occur in the brain, called *dopamine and norepinephrine*. Previously, doctors tried elevating her serotonin, which provided no improvement, but they never tried elevating her dopamine or norepinephrine levels.

I asked her to tell me about AD/HD, and when she did, I could see myself in the criteria, even though I had been a teacher for over twenty years. After being carefully screened, I, too, was diagnosed with AD/HD. I wondered how many other fibromyalgia or other patients with chronic pain might fit the AD/HD criteria. If so, would treatment improve their symptoms like it had mine?

Overcoming the Problems

Fortunately, Glenda Davis, MD, diagnosed me with AD/HD, and she was already aware of the AD/HD and FMS connection. However, most doctors do not know of the connection between these disorders, and many are not open to exploring the connection because of the absence of double-blind studies.

Another problem is that stimulants are illegal for any condition other than AD/HD or narcolepsy. That means you must meet AD/HD criteria and be diagnosed with AD/HD to be eligible to use stimulant medications, which help balance dopamine and norepinephrine. However, there are other medications that affect dopamine, like pramipexole and bupropion, which can be used without an AD/HD diagnosis.

Improper dosing of medications and supplements that affect dopamine is a common error made in treatment. When the dosage is too low, benefits do not occur. Too much can make you feel worse, but the right amount of the right medication can dramatically improve health and well-being. I believe most patients and many doctors who work with medications that affect dopamine do not know how important correct dosing can be. One possible reason for this is most doctors have used stimulant medications that affect dopamine and norepinephrine mainly on children with AD/HD. Perhaps children are incapable of providing good feedback in order to help the doctor fine-tune the dosage.

I see basically the same thing in supplements that affect dopamine, but not to the same degree. When using supplements that affect dopamine, *dosage is very important to ensure benefit.* In other words, most clients start low and work their way up until they see benefit.

Not all supplements and medications that affect dopamine and norepinephrine will benefit all patients equally. One supplement or medication might work better for one patient than another. Usually, the first one works, but not always.

SPECT Scan Shows Similarities between FMS and AD/HD

I had a SPECT Scan (monitors blood flowing into the brain) done previously by fibromyalgia researchers in Birmingham, Alabama (USA). It showed insufficient blood flow into the frontal lobes of my brain, which was consistent with other fibromyalgia patients. I sent this scan to an AD/HD researcher at Emory in Atlanta, Georgia (USA). She told me that they see this same blood flow pattern in AD/HD patients.

Getting the Word Out

Years before I knew anything about natural medicine, I started talking with many other fibromyalgia patients, after I found profound relief. Most also believed they fit the AD/HD criteria, a condition with generally low dopamine and other brain chemicals, not just now, but all their lives.

I shared my story and my research with many of the doctors who had seen my "before" and "after," only to find them uninterested in what had helped me. This disturbed me to the point that I felt I had to share with a larger audience.

Other Considerations

In 1998, I began hosting a Web site regarding a connection between fibromyalgia and AD/HD. The many letters I received from this Web site reinforced my belief about this connection. Also, after talking to people in my locality with FMS, I have also seen many gain dramatic relief with AD/HD medications.

Another reason why this connection can be important is this medical approach is covered under most insurance policies. Natural supplements are out-of-pocket expenses, and many cannot afford them. Therefore, cost can be a factor in the approach chosen.

Melanie

When I first met Melanie about twelve years ago, before I began my work with natural medicine, she was a high school student with fibromyalgia. She was struggling to finish school because of the FMS pain. She and her mother sat down with me. I shared my recovery using AD/HD medications and balancing hormones. At first, Melanie did not see herself in the AD/HD criteria, but her mother spoke up and said other close family members fit the AD/HD criteria. I recommended that she see a psychiatrist I knew. She was evaluated and treated for AD/HD. The medication stopped her pain rather quickly. She successfully completed high school and college and was pain free the last time I talked to her several years later. Other family members were also diagnosed and treated.

AD/HD can be Difficult to Diagnose

The hallmark symptoms of AD/HD are inattention, impulsivity, and hyperactivity,[73] but no two with AD/HD are exactly alike. *Many do not have the hyperactive component.* There is no blood test or other way to measure AD/HD currently. The diagnosis is based on a thorough evaluation by a knowledgeable clinician.

Adults can be more difficult to diagnose with AD/HD because we have learned to compensate. We are often intelligent enough to work around our weaknesses, but years of compensation can take a toll on us emotionally and physically. However, when most adults who have AD/HD see the diagnostic criteria, we understand that it fits us. But some who fit the AD/HD criteria, based on another family member's evaluation, do not see it themselves. It is also easy to think that AD/HD is normal because we are born with it and it tends to run in our families. Often our family members have similar tendencies, so it may be "normal" within the family. It is thought to be a biological condition, most often inherited.[74]

Flaws of the AD/HD Criteria in Adults and Problems with Diagnosis

Some physicians question the validity of using traditional AD/HD criteria for adult patients. Only in recent years have more adults come forward to be screened for AD/HD. In the past, physicians thought children outgrew AD/HD. Many adults, including me, will tell you this is not true.

Kathleen Nadeau, PhD, and Patricia Quinn, MD, in their book *Understanding Women with AD/HD*, state, "There is increasing agreement among experts in the field [of ADHD] that the DSM-IV criteria used to diagnose AD/HD are not entirely appropriate for adults, and perhaps even less appropriate for women."[75] The AD/HD criteria (DSM-IV-TR) most doctors use is designed and used predominately for children because most who have been diagnosed with AD/HD are children. However, more relevant diagnostic criteria are being developed for adults because of the growing awareness that adults can also have AD/HD. Often, this is discovered when they are in the doctor's office with their own children.

So where do adults interested in this connection begin? They need to consider the finer points of AD/HD such as in the book, *Understanding Women with AD/HD* by Kathleen Nadeau, PhD, and Patricia Quinn, MD, or *Driven to Distraction* by Edward Hallowell, MD, and John Ratey, MD. If they see themselves in the criteria, they can make notes from each criterion, find a doctor who treats *adult* AD/HD, and ask to be screened for AD/HD. Before going in, they should also write a page summarizing specific examples throughout their lives that demonstrate points of the AD/HD criteria. They could also take a family member to also share his/her perspective.

Diagnostic criteria are listed at the end of this chapter.

Links are listed at the end of the chapter to explore AD/HD.

Neurotransmitter Imbalances

Edward Hallowell, MD, and John Ratey, MD, state in their book *Driven to Distraction* that "no single neurotransmitter system may be the sole regulator of ADD. The most likely possibility is that the effect of dopamine and norepinephrine and serotonin is key and drugs that alter these neurotransmitters will have the most telling effect on the symptoms of ADD."[76] [ADD now is often referred to as AD/HD.] This is an important quote.

The Possible Stress Factor in AD/HD and FMS

A significant amount of women find they are bombarded with the responsibilities of caring for their families, housework, errands, working outside the home, and community or church activities. This can create chronic stress. Also, growing up with AD/HD can create stresses of its own. Many children with AD/HD report disruptive home lives, which contributes to the stress.

According to Jerry Lithman, MD and Gail Rodin, PhD, "All three variables—genetic vulnerability, early exposure to highly stressful situations, and current stress level—are associated with the risk of developing FMS.[77]

Daniel Amen, MD also states, "Fibromyalgia and ADD commonly coexist. I think the chronic stress associated with ADD is in part responsible for the muscle pain."[78]

Dispelling the Misconceptions

After talking with thousands of adults about AD/HD through my Web site, I learned that most adults really do not understand what AD/HD really is. To dispel some of the misconceptions, AD/HD is *not* always associated with:

1. a lack of intelligence
2. low achievement
3. difficulty getting through school
4. hyperactivity

This can make diagnosis more difficult. All with AD/HD do not necessarily display all symptoms of AD/HD. Some people have mild AD/HD and others have it more severely.[79]

Conventional Treatment Options

Adults with AD/HD frequently have coexisting disorders, such as depression, manic depression (bipolar), or anxiety. Sometimes these respond to the stimulant alone. However, they may need an antidepressant [which affects serotonin] and a stimulant, [which affects dopamine] (primarily beta activity] and norepinephrine [alpha and beta activity]. Balancing these chemicals can be critical to success.

Stimulant medications are treatment of choice for AD/HD. These medications are controlled substances, which means they are tightly managed. Each prescription must be hand written. They cannot be called in. You must be diagnosed with AD/HD or narcolepsy (sleeping attacks) in order to gain access to stimulant medications.

I challenge you to carefully consider the information in this chapter, and even if you "know" you do not have AD/HD, you might humbly ask a loved one to evaluate you, since others see us more objectively. Even if you have AD/HD, you do not necessarily need to treat it. You might want to if it is compromising your quality of life.

Patricia Stephens, C.N.C

Dispelling the Fear of AD/HD Medications

Even though I am far from being an authority on AD/HD medications, what I will present here is something you can do further research on. What I have learned concerning these medications has come from my own personal experience, doctors who have taken time to teach me, listening to others I have come in contact with personally, and responses from my old Web site www.addfibro.com, and a great deal of personal research on the subject of AD/HD.

After working in a natural pharmacy for ten years, I listen to the fears of some parents and adults who either have AD/HD children or see it in themselves. Often I hear them tell me they are fearful about becoming addicted to or harmed by these medications.

> The research so far suggests that individuals with AD/HD *do not become addicted* to their stimulant medications when taken in the form and dosage prescribed by their doctors. And there have been several studies that report stimulant therapy in childhood does *not* increase the risk for subsequent drug and alcohol abuse.[80]

Even thought I am extremely sensitive, I had no negative side effects with the right dosage of stimulant. I also had no withdrawal when I stopped using it.

The book *Images into the Mind*, written by Daniel Amen, MD, a respected psychiatrist and AD/HD researcher, dispels fears about addiction in using low-dose stimulants to treat AD/HD. I watched the video version of it years ago and haven't forgotten the powerful images and information he presented.

From my own experience using stimulant medications and after talking to a large group of others who use them, I know that side effects can occur, but, almost without exception, they occur when the dosage is incorrect. Often, just a small adjustment in dosage can stop a negative side effect. Sometimes, one medication will work better for someone than another, but most of the time the first medication works.

Finding and Working with a Medical Professional

Most of the time, it is best to locate a psychiatrist. Generally, they work more with AD/HD medications and understand how to correctly dose them. Many psychologists diagnose AD/HD, but they cannot write a prescription. However, they can refer you, and their referral counts a lot. Many psychologists also understand how to work with the medications. Some family practitioners work with AD/HD patients and are good at balancing AD/HD medications. Occasionally other doctors might work with stimulant medications, but it is out of the ordinary.

If, after reading the AD/HD criteria at the end of this chapter, you see yourself and want to pursue this, here are some important tips to consider before locating a physician.

1. If you are trying to locate a physician, you could call a local pharmacist to see who treats adult AD/HD locally. Because they fill prescriptions, they should know which doctors write prescriptions for AD/HD medications. They might also be aware of the reputation of doctors who prescribe. CHADD, which is an organization

formed to provide education, advocacy, and support for children and adults with attention deficit/hyperactivity disorder, can help.

2. If you fit the AD/HD criteria, write a page of examples in your life showing how the criteria specifically fit you.

3. From the time you enter your doctor's office, mention that you would like to be screened for AD/HD in the *first three minutes* before your doctor puts you in another preconceived diagnosis. (A psychiatrist once told me this. I believed him.)

4. Remember that proper dosing of medication is critical to success. It is the most common error made in treating AD/HD. Medications work best when you are using the right dosage for your body.

5. Stimulants are the medication of choice for AD/HD. Other medications can help, but stimulants are the mainstay.

6. Sometimes more than one medication is needed for adult AD/HD patients, such as a stimulant and an antidepressant.

7. Know that AD/HD medications are legal only for AD/HD and narcolepsy. Most doctors are unaware of a connection between FMS and AD/HD. If you fit the AD/HD criteria, ask to be screened for AD/HD. (You might not want to mention FMS because it is not their area of expertise and you might scare off your doctor. Focus on the AD/HD.)

8. Be prepared to work with the dosage of your medications. Your doctor should be able to assist you in getting the dosage correct. This can be very easy, or it can take some persistence.

CHADD organizations throughout the country usually help patients find a knowledgeable physician who works with adult AD/HD. www.chadd.org

Fibromyalgia and Attention Deficit/ Hyperactivity Disorder

Other professionals, such as Jerry Lithman, MD, and Gail Rodin, PhD., have also seen a connection between AD/HD and fibromyalgia:

> We have worked with many individuals with ADHD, FMS, or both disorders. Our experience has led up to believe that there are links between ADHD and FMS and that it is especially important to women with ADHD to understand these links in order to remain healthy.[81]
>
> We believe that a cornerstone for the prevention and treatment of FMS is the recognition of underlying ADHD and initiation of its treatment with medication (usually a psychostimulant) that effects the necessary redistribution of monoamine neurotransmitters (*dopamine*, norepinephrine, and serotonin).[82]
>
> —Lithman, Rodin,
> *Understanding Women with ADHD*

If fibromyalgia patients are diagnosed with AD/HD, I believe it is very important to start with a medication that is not timed-released. You cannot cut time-released products up to find the right dosage that is so critical to well-being. After finding the right dosage, then you will likely be able to find a time-released product that might work just as well for you. Remember the rule. The right medication, taken in the right amount, taken at the right time of the day can "turn lights on in very dark rooms."

Hormonal Involvement

Women often find that the amount of medication they take often needs adjusting at certain times of their menstrual cycle. Glenda Davis, MD, taught me that many women have to go up or down on their stimulant medication often just a couple days before their period to keep their chemistry smooth. With their doctor's permission, it is usually better to decrease it first as a trial. If that is not effective, they may need to increase their dosage at certain times of their cycle for smoothness in treatment.

Many other studies have been done on the effects of hormonal imbalance and brain performance. According to Patricia Quinn, MD, "Estrogen and progesterone seem to have both direct and indirect central nervous system effects. In addition, it is becoming clearer that these hormones can also affect the response of psychostimulants."[83]

Memory and Hormones

"Estrogen was also shown to enhance both short and long term memory and the capacity to learn new associations. Estrogen helps maintain verbal memory and enhances the capacity for new learning in women."[84] [85] "As estrogen levels fall, beginning at perimenopause and continuing into menopause, brain volume in females begins to decline. This atrophy occurs mainly in the hippocampus and the parietal lobe, areas primarily associated with memory and cognition."[86] [87]

Natural Alternatives

Medications are not the only option, although conventional medications are usually more powerful, at least initially. Plants can be very helpful. Many of these support concentration and focus and decrease hyperactivity. Many children and adults achieve good results with alternative treatments. *In the end, what matters most is what works best.*

There are many products on the market which combine supplements. *Often combining plants enhances effectiveness.*

In general, children (age six to twelve) usually take half the adult dosage. Remember that dosages matter and they vary widely. Work the dosage carefully before switching to a different supplement.

Supplements That Can Support Calm Focus

Fish Oil

Fish oil supports better memory and mood. Unknowingly, lowering dietary fat intake can create a deficiency of fatty acids necessary for normal brain functioning. Many of us eat the wrong kinds of fats. Fish oil has a variety of other benefits, which are addressed in the "Lifestyle Changes" chapter. [Use caution when purchasing fish oil. Inexpensive fish oils might not be pure. Better fish oils are "distilled" or "molecularly distilled" to ensure there is no mercury contamination.] Most use 2,000 to 4,000 milligrams daily with a meal. Remember, children generally use half the adult dosage.

Patricia Stephens, C.N.C

Phosphatidylserine

Phosphatidylserine often is available in combination with other supplements, but it is effective by itself. It can improve sleep, focus and concentration, mood and energy. Most use 100 milligrams one to three times daily. Adults and children benefit from using phosphatidylserine, which is commonly referred to as PS.

SAM-e (S-adenosyl methionine)

I have seen impressive changes in clients through the years with SAM-e. Some of the benefits are better mood in about a week, improved energy, and less pain over the course of five to six weeks.

Dr. Quinn and Dr. Nadeau state, "SAM-e remains an intriguing alternative for refractory [does not respond to traditional therapy] AD/HD or in some women with co-morbid [more than one diagnosis] depression. Although appealing, SAM-e has not been studied under controlled conditions for the treatment of AD/HD."[88]

Most start SAM-e with 200 milligrams twice daily on an empty stomach. In a few days to a week, if no benefit is noted, they increase the dosage to 400 milligrams twice daily. A few have to increase up to 800 milligrams two times daily. As soon as benefit is noticed, often the dosage can be reduced to 200 milligrams twice daily for maintenance.

Dr. Daniel Amen, a well-known psychiatrist, author of the book *Healing ADD*, states that SAM-e is helpful for ADD because many important brain chemicals are produced from SAM-e. "SAM-e is one of the best natural antidepressants available, and a number of studies have shown that it is as effective as antidepressant medications. SAM-e has also been found helpful for people who suffer from fibromyalgia.

Do not use SAM-e if you have been diagnosed with manic-depression (bipolar), unless advised by a medical professional.

NADH (nicotinamide adenine dinucleotide)

NADH works at the cellular level to facilitate the conversion of glucose to energy. It is used widely to improve memory, concentration, and mood. Many clients also receive pain relief from NADH when the dosage is correct. It often works quickly but can take up to six weeks to note improvement.

Most begin NADH by taking 2.5 milligrams once a day on an empty stomach (thirty minutes before a meal). In a few days, if no change, increasing the dosage can make a significant difference. Many use 5 to 20 milligrams daily.

Most find the benefits of NADH last all day. There are few side effects noted with it, as long as the dosage is not too high. Insomnia could be a sign that the dosage is too high.

Often NADH needs to be combined with something, like SAM-e or St. John's Wort, for greatest benefit, but not always.

L-Theanine

Many benefit greatly from L-theanine. It often works quickly to calm anxiety and improve focus and concentration. Dosage is often 50 to 100 milligrams two to three times daily.

Patricia Stephens, C.N.C

St. John's Wort

Dr. Amen uses St. John's Wort for his patients with depression and over-focus issues. He states, "The starting dosage of St. John's Wort is 300 mg a day for children, 300 mg. twice a day for teens, and 600 mg in the morning and 300 mg. at night for adults."[89] It is recommended not to combine it with conventional antidepressant medications. It can take three weeks or more to provide benefits.

Gingko

Gingko is one of the oldest known supplements. It has been used for hundreds of years to assist blood flow to the brain, which can facilitate improved concentration and mood. Most find that it works within six weeks. The dosage is often 60 to 180 milligrams daily.

GABA (Gamma-aminobutyric acid)

GABA is thought to be one of the most important neurotransmitters in the central nervous system. It promotes calm, tranquil feelings, which can reduce hyperactivity and improve focus. It can help those with temper problems, anxiety, and irritability. Dosage range varies from 100 milligrams daily and up for adults and generally half that dosage for children.

Newer forms of GABA, such as Pharma GABA, cross the blood brain-barrier much more effectively, rendering more noticeable improvements.

DL-phenylalanine-(DLPA)

DLPA is an amino acid that aids in the production of norepinephrine. It improves depression, pain relief, and energy. The dosage range is 500 milligrams one to three times daily, although some take more. It works best on an empty stomach.

Multivitamin

Many children are not getting enough nutrition from their diets. A good multivitamin can provide benefit to adults and children with AD/HD.

Summary

- If you think you fit the AD/HD criteria and are interested in pursuing conventional treatment, write down how you specifically fit the criteria.

- Find a professional in your area experienced in working with AD/HD. A local CHADD organization or local pharmacist can often help you locate a professional. You might also do some internet research.

- Mention AD/HD early in the appointment. This is very important.

- The right amount of the right medication at the right time of day will foster the greatest improvements. Be prepared to work with the medications. You may not feel or function better until you are close to your maintenance dosage.

- If you are perimenopausal or postmenopausal, hormonal imbalances can be contributing factors to your symptoms.

Most doctors are unaware of a connection between fibromyalgia and AD/HD. If you see yourself in the

AD/HD criteria and you choose medical treatment, know that a doctor must diagnose you with AD/HD before he/she can prescribe a stimulant medication. As your AD/HD is treated correctly, your FMS symptoms will probably improve dramatically. Perhaps other chronic complaints will also respond when brain chemistry is balanced.

Important Note: Web addresses sometimes change. If you cannot locate the web address below, you can enter a name or topic on a Internet search engine in order to locate it.

Resources

Two of the best books that I have seen on adult female AD/HD are compiled by Kathleen Nadeau, PhD, and Patricia Quinn, MD. The first is a patient-directed book entitled *Understanding Women with ADHD*. The second book, *Gender Issues in ADHD Women*, is focused more toward physicians. They host an impressive Web site regarding female AD/HD at www.addvance.com.

Glenda H. Davis, MD has a Web site with excellent information regarding the connection between fibromyalgia and AD/HD www.sounddoctrin.com.

At the time of this writing, Daniel Amen, MD has a wonderful Web site with excellent information on AD/HD. The link sited has a good test including the finer points of the disorder. www.amenclinic.com/ac/test/add_test1.php

Dr. Amen also has some excellent, detailed

information on supplements in AD/HD patients: http://amenclinics.com/bp/articles.php?articleID=10

Another good Web site is hosted by Dr. Carol Watkins and other medical professionals. She has interesting information on women with AD/HD. www.ncpamd.com/Girls_Women_AD/HD.htm

CHADD (Children and adults with attention deficit hyperactivity disorder) www.chadd.org

The following AD/HD criteria is the official one used by clinicians to make a diagnosis of AD/HD.

ADHD Criteria

DSM-IV Diagnostic Criteria for ADHD

The year 2000 Diagnostic and Statistical Manual for Mental Disorders (DSM-IV-TR) provides criteria for diagnosing ADHD.

The year 2000 Diagnostic & Statistical Manual for Mental Disorders (DSM-IV-TR) provides criteria for diagnosing AD/HD. The criteria are presented here in modified form in order to make them more accessible to the general public. They are listed here for information purposes and should be used only by trained health care providers to diagnose or treat AD/HD.

DSM-IV Criteria for AD/HD

I. Either A or B:

    A. Six or more of the following symptoms of inattention have been present for at least 6 months to a point that is disruptive and inappropriate for developmental level:

Inattention

    1. Often does not give close attention to details or makes careless mistakes in schoolwork, work, or other activities.

2. Often has trouble keeping attention on tasks or play activities.

3. Often does not seem to listen when spoken to directly.

4. Often does not follow instructions and fails to finish schoolwork, chores, or duties in the workplace (not due to oppositional behavior or failure to understand instructions).

5. Often has trouble organizing activities.

6. Often avoids, dislikes, or doesn't want to do things that take a lot of mental effort for a long period of time (such as schoolwork or homework).

7. Often loses things needed for tasks and activities (e.g. toys, school assignments, pencils, books, or tools).

8. Is often easily distracted.

9. Is often forgetful in daily activities.

B. Six or more of the following symptoms of hyperactivity-impulsivity have been present for at least 6 months to an extent that is disruptive and inappropriate for developmental level:

Hyperactivity

1. Often fidgets with hands or feet or squirms in seat.

2. Often gets up from seat when remaining in seat is expected.

3. Often runs about or climbs when and where it is not appropriate (adolescents or adults may feel very restless).

4. Often has trouble playing or enjoying leisure activities quietly.

5. Is often "on the go" or often acts as if "driven by a motor".

6. Often talks excessively.

Impulsivity

1. Often blurts out answers before questions have been finished.

2. Often has trouble waiting one's turn.

3. Often interrupts or intrudes on others (e.g., butts into conversations or games).

II. Some symptoms that cause impairment were present before age 7 years.

III. Some impairment from the symptoms is present in two or more settings (e.g. at school/work and at home).

IV. There must be clear evidence of significant impairment in social, school, or work functioning.

V. The symptoms do not happen only during the course of a Pervasive Developmental Disorder, Schizophrenia, or other Psychotic Disorder. The symptoms are not better accounted for by another mental disorder (e.g. Mood Disorder, Anxiety Disorder, Dissociative Disorder, or a Personality Disorder).

Based on these criteria, three types of AD/HD are identified:

1. AD/HD, *Combined Type*: if both criteria 1A and 1B are met for the past 6 months

2. AD/HD, *Predominantly Inattentive Type*: if criterion 1A is met but criterion 1B is not met for the past six months

3. AD/HD, *Predominantly Hyperactive-Impulsive*

Patricia Stephens, C.N.C

Type: if Criterion 1B is met but Criterion 1A is not met for the past six months.

American Psychiatric Association: Diagnostic and Statistical Manual of Mental Disorders, Fourth Edition, Text Revision. Washington, DC, American Psychiatric Association, 2000.

Glenda H. Davis, MD, has developed criteria used in conjunction with the DSM-IV-TR criteria when screening patients for AD/HD. She gave permission to include it. This describes some of the finer points.

Mood/Behavior Questionnaire
MBQ-R2007 Glenda Hawkins Davis, MD

Name: _____

Age: _____ Date: ____/____/____

Yes No Do you:

1. ( ) ( ) Often have trouble sitting still? (fidgety, shifting a lot, wiggling foot, etc.)

2. ( ) ( ) Often feel nervous or restless inside, even when everything is going well?

3. ( ) ( ) Often miss important details or make careless mistakes?

4. ( ) ( ) Often bite your nails or chew on things (gum, pens, clothes, etc.)?

5. ( ) ( ) Often get easily distracted by things going on around you?

6. ( ) ( ) Often take longer than others to eat, bathe, or dress?

7. ( ) ( ) Often has difficulty understanding or following directions?

8. ( ) ( ) Often have difficulty waiting or get very impatient while waiting?

9. ( ) ( ) Often have difficulty finishing what you start?

10. ( ) ( ) Often get bored easily?

11. ( ) ( ) Often talk too much?

12. ( ) ( ) Often hurt others' feelings without meaning to?

13. ( ) ( ) Often get your feelings hurt easily?

14. ( ) ( ) Often get irritated or angry easily?

15. ( ) ( ) Often get emotional or cry easily over others' problems?

16. ( ) ( ) Often dislike the way clothes feel on you (wrong texture, too tight, too loose)?

17. ( ) ( ) Often get upset over things not being even or symmetrical?

18. ( ) ( ) Often get upset over changes in your routine?

19. ( ) ( ) Often interrupt when others are talking?

20. ( ) ( ) Often finish others' sentences for them?

21. ( ) ( ) Often answer a question before it is completely asked?

22. ( ) ( ) Often "tune out" or not listen when others are talking to you (not intentionally)?

23. ( ) ( ) Often daydream when you should be listening?

Patricia Stephens, C.N.C

24. ( ) ( ) Often forget things that are important to you (appointments, occasions, etc.)?

25. ( ) ( ) Often lose or misplace things?

26. ( ) ( ) Often get accused of doing things that you really don't think you did?

27. ( ) ( ) Often have trouble getting unimportant things off your mind (tune, incident)

28. ( ) ( ) Often get into trouble even when you are trying to do right?

29. ( ) ( ) Often do just enough to "get by" instead of doing your best?

30. ( ) ( ) Often get upset with yourself over things you do or say?

31. ( ) ( ) Often get upset with others for things they do or say?

32. ( ) ( ) Often feel like a failure?

33. ( ) ( ) Often feel like giving up?

34. ( ) ( ) Often feel like others would be better off if you were not around?

35. ( ) ( ) Often feel overwhelmed with life or with what others expect of you?

36. ( ) ( ) Often feel tired or sleepy during the day?

37. ( ) ( ) Often have trouble sleeping (can't go to sleep, or awaken during the night)?

38. ( ) ( ) Often have trouble staying awake when sitting still (in the car, in church, etc.)?

39. ( ) ( ) Often eat when you are not hungry (when bored, upset, worried, etc.)?

40. ( ) ( )   Often put things off until
the last minute?

41. ( ) ( )   Often have trouble getting organized to
do things (getting materials together)?

42. ( ) ( )   Often smoke, or drink alcohol, or caf-
feine to calm you down or pick you up?

43. ( ) ( )   Often do careless or danger-
ous things without think-
ing about the consequences?

44. ( ) ( )   Often bump into things or
knock things over?

45. ( ) ( )   Often feel very disorganized?

46. ( ) ( )   Often allow yourself to com-
mit to too many things at once
and get overwhelmed?

47. ( ) ( )   Often misjudge the amount of time you
need to do something or get somewhere?

48. ( ) ( )   Often show extremes of messi-
ness (room, desk, car, etc.)?

49. ( ) ( )   Often show extremes of neatness (everything has to be in its exact place)?

50. ( ) ( )   Often take longer than others to complete tasks?

51. ( ) ( )   Often rush through your work?

52. ( ) ( )   Often feel as if you are always in a
hurry or in "high gear" or behind?

53. ( ) ( )   Often misunderstand what is said
in conversations or jokes?

54. ( ) ( )   Often feel "picked on" or unloved?

55. ( ) ( ) Often have headaches?

56. ( ) ( ) Often have stomach trouble?

57. ( ) ( ) Often have diarrhea when under stress?

58. ( ) ( ) Often have trouble with constipation?

59. ( ) ( ) Often have sweaty feet and/or hands?

60. ( ) ( ) Often have cold feet and/or hands?

61. ( ) ( ) Often have itchy skin or skin rashes?

62. ( ) ( ) Often find it difficult to *not*
pick at sores or scabs?

63. ( ) ( ) Often have tremors—shaky hands?

64. ( ) ( ) Often feel hotter or colder
than those around you?

65. ( ) ( ) Often have stiff or achy muscles?

66. ( ) ( ) Often get dizzy when you
stand up quickly?

67. ( ) ( ) Often feel unmotivated to do anything?

68. ( ) ( ) Often get physically tired when standing?

69. ( ) ( ) Often get very enthusiastic about a
project but quickly lose interest?

70. ( ) ( ) Often feel uncomfortable when
your surroundings are too quiet?

71. ( ) ( ) Often feel uncomfortable when
your surroundings are too noisy?

72. ( ) ( ) Often concentrate best with back-
ground noise (TV, radio, etc.)?

73. ( ) ( ) Often concentrate best with no noise?

74. ( ) ( ) Often get distracted even when alone?

75. ( ) ( ) Often have to read things over and over to get the full meaning?

76. ( ) ( ) Often have trouble getting along with people in authority?

77. ( ) ( ) Often have trouble tolerating others' mistakes?

Note: Everyone has some of these symptoms. No one has all of them. The key word is *often*—is this *characteristic* of you? If you want to check "sometimes," you may put a check between yes and no.

Glenda H. Davis, MD
Web site: www.sounddoctrin.com

Dopamine And Norepinephrine: Overlooked, Important Brain Chemicals

An important relationship exists between low dopamine levels and chronic complaints, including pain. For the most part, this connection has virtually gone unnoticed. Improving my own dopamine, norepinephrine, and serotonin levels completely resolved my chronic pain and other chronic complaints. For me, balancing brain chemicals and hormones has provided long-term benefits. I have seen these same improvements in too many others to ignore this connection. For years, I could not find this connection in print, but finally good medical documentation is surfacing.

Lessons That Evolved

After observing substantial improvements in fibromyalgia sufferers, I believe the connection between up-regulating dopamine in chronically ill patients must be addressed and studied. Who better to do this than the medical community? Perhaps patients will take this message to their doctors.

Even though stimulant medications worked so well for me years ago, I have not used these medications in ten years, and I remain pain-free. There are many ways to elevate brain chemicals. One way to balance brain chemicals can be by balancing hormones. Sometimes that is enough to improve brain chemical production. Other times supplements or medications are needed to regulate brain chemistry.

A Relationship between Hormones and Brain Chemicals

Elizabeth Vliet, MD, discusses the important role brain chemicals play, including serotonin, norepinephrine, dopamine, acetylcholine, and gamma amino butyric acid (GABA), all of which influence mood and physical symptoms. She emphasizes the link between the brain chemicals and hormones: "These molecules function to convey and modulate information going back and forth between the brain and the body. They provide an important link between emotional and physical health."[90]

As you can see from Dr. Vliet's comments, it is hard to separate the benefits of hormones from neurotransmitters because their work is tightly intertwined.

I have noticed impressive mood changes in myself and clients when hormones are balanced. Balanced hormones have often produced dramatic reduction or eradication of physical complaints. I have observed other women besides myself who are able to get off psychiatric medications when hormones are balanced.

Antidepressants: Standard Treatment Protocol

When I was going from doctor to doctor looking for answers for my chronic health problems, the standard protocol was to put patients on antidepressants. After trying many different ones, I found them completely ineffective, or they caused such bad side effects I could not tolerate them.

Most doctors who treat fibromyalgia patients and other chronic-pain patients recognize the need to treat low serotonin levels, which is the brain chemical many antidepressants affect. Yet most patients have only limited success using SSRI antidepressants. Few doctors are aware of problems that can surface when the neurotransmitter dopamine becomes unbalanced. Correcting this chemical imbalance can quickly and dramatically improve our quality of life, especially when it is balanced with norepinephrine and serotonin.

Dopamine Research

Dr. Patrick Wood, MD, a fibromyalgia researcher at the LSU Health Science Center in Shreveport, Louisiana, states, "Boosting serotonin in patients with chronic widespread pain has met with limited success insofar as analgesia (pain relief) is concerned."[91]

He is doing impressive research currently on dopamine and fibromyalgia. This research has caught the eye of the National Fibromyalgia Association. He states, "A growing body of evidence exists to suggest that the pain of fibromyalgia may stem from a deregulation of dopamine neurotransmission in brain centers in which dopamine plays a role in natural analgesia [pain relief], most of which fall into the domain of the greater limbic system."[92] The implications for future therapies for fibromyalgia, and indeed many other chronic pain conditions, are discussed in light of these insights.[93]

I interpret this to mean that correcting these imbalances in neurotransmitters can improve fibromyalgia and other chronic-pain syndromes.

Another doctor who has seen improvements in fibromyalgia (FMS) patients by increasing dopamine is Dr. Andrew J. Holman. He is a rheumatologist and researcher who has published studies on using a medication called pramipexole in fibromyalgia patients. This medication affects dopamine. He states, "In a subset of patients with fibromyalgia, roughly fifty percent of the FMS patients in the study who used pramipexole had improved scores on assessments of pain, fatigue, function, and global status, and [it] was safe and well-tolerated."[94]

Other Medical Documentation

Elizabeth Vliet, MD, also has seen the benefits of elevating dopamine and other neurotransmitters in chronically ill patients. She states, "In addition to overlooking the role of female hormones in fibromyalgia, we have also been too slow in looking at some of the brain hormones and chemical messengers (serotonin, dopamine, epinephrine, substance p, and others) in approaching chronic pain as a problem very different from acute pain." [95]

Another FMS researcher using medications to improve dopamine and serotonin is Daniel Malone, MD, a rheumatologist at the University of Wisconsin. He has been treating FMS patients with a combina-

Patricia Stephens, C.N.C

tion of dopaminergic and serotonergic drugs including L-dopa, 5-HTP, fenfluramine, pemoline and phentermine. He found statistical improvement in 76 patients out of 122 using this method. Unfortunately, two of the medications he had been using, fenfluramine and phentermine, have been withdrawn from the market because of serious heart-valve complications found in some patients taking these medications for weight loss.[96] Also Pemoline (Cylert) is rarely used because of required liver function tests every two weeks.

A group of German physicians also have seen benefits in fibromyalgia patients after using AD/HD medications. Dr. K. Krause, J. Krause, Magyarosy, Ernst, and Pongratz state, "In our clinical experience with adult patients with attention deficit/hyperactivity disorder (AD/HD) some patients experienced relief of concomitant fibromyalgia complaints by medication for therapy of AD/HD like methylphenidate (generic Ritalin)."[97]

Stimulants, like methylphenidate (Ritalin), enhance dopamine and norepinephrine, chemicals naturally occurring in the brain.

Supplements Which Affect Dopamine and Other Brain Chemicals

Many plant-based supplements that affect dopamine also affect other brain chemicals. Nature has a way of creating a balance.

I have seen the following supplements benefit clients. I have listed them somewhat in priority order. However, individuals may respond much better to one supplement than another. Proper dosing can be critical to success.

NADH (nicotinamide adenine dinucleotide)
(The *H* stands for hydrogen.)

Some fibromyalgia patients respond well to a supplement called NADH which helps increase dopamine, serotonin, and norepinephrine. It often works, but the dosage has to be right. Most start low and work their way up until they feel better.

Dr. Jacob Teitelbaum, Medical Director of the Fibromyalgia Centers discusses the importance of NADH in his book, *From Fatigue to Fantastic:*

> In people with FMS/CFIDS the body has difficulty producing NADH. Because NADH has many other functions, a lack of it is disastrous for the body. One major function of NADH is in stimulating the production of important neurotransmitters dopamine, norepinephrine, and serotonin. Serotonin is important for sleep and emotional balance. Norepinephrine is responsible for alertness, concentration, and mental activity. Dopamine is also responsible for a sense of well-being, and for energizing the body. It stimulates strength, coordination, cognition (mental functioning), mood, sex drive and the secretion of growth hormone, which is also low in people with FMS/Chronic Fatigue Immune Dysfunction Syndrome. These neurotransmitters appear to be low in people with FMS/CFIDS. [98]
>
> —Teitelbaum, *From Fatigue to Fantastic*

I have used NADH successfully in FMS/CFS clients. I recommend my clients start with 5 milligrams once a day on an empty stomach. After a few days, if they see no change, I tell them to go up to 10 milligrams a day. Usually this dosage works, and it usually works in a couple of days. However, occasionally it takes longer to become effective. Research shows it can take up to six weeks. If the dose is high enough, it usually works much faster, but not always. Some people may need to take it twice a day. There are also some who need a very small dosage. When someone is sensitive, I start them with 2.5 milligrams.

Jane

Jane told me she wanted a natural alternative to a stimulant. We discussed NADH, and she decided to try it for her FMS symptoms. She emailed me and said, "I did try NADH yesterday. For the nine hours it was active in my system, it was a miracle. I was clear-headed, alert, and intelligent for the first time in years. Plus, I was calm and not at all hyper or 'speedy.' While I was clear-headed, I did some research on it and discovered the dopamine connection." She goes on to say when the NADH wears off, her symptoms return.

I have seen many clients use NADH with conventional antidepressants without problem. Many FMS patients benefit from NADH alone, while others need to add 5 HTP, St. John's Wort, or SAM-e for optimal benefit.

SAM-e

SAM-e may relieve pain in fibromyalgia and arthritis patients. It can improve mood within a week but may take up to six weeks to see pain relief. I start clients with 200 milligrams twice a day on an *empty stomach*.

Often it is not effective at this dosage. Some clients require 400 to 800 milligrams two to three times a day. Once improvement is seen, patients can try dropping to about 200 milligrams twice a day. A very few have reported stomach distress with SAM-e, which usually passes after a few days. Also, decreasing the dosage can correct the problem. Purchasing a quality product is also important.

FMS patients using SAM-e have shown significant improvement in pain reduction, according to a study done by Dr. Tavoni and colleagues.

Those who did not improve may not have been taking enough SAM-e. Also they might have seen more improvement if they had taken it with NADH for maximum effectiveness. Often combining products makes a significant difference.

Although SAM-e is expensive, most clients find it is worth its cost. Because of its expense, I often try other supplements first in clients. It should not be taken with conventional antidepressants without your doctor's permission. It is not recommended in patients diagnosed with manic-depression (bipolar disorder).

5 HTP (5 Hydroxytryptophan)

The supplement 5 HTP has been shown to be very effective in the treatment of fibromyalgia and other chronic-pain conditions. The proposed mechanism of action is that 5 HTP increases levels of serotonin, melatonin, norepinephrine, and dopamine.

Three clinical trials have demonstrated significant improvements in symptoms, including pain, morning stiffness, anxiety, and fatigue.[100] [101] [102] Patients also report improved sleep and headache relief with

Patricia Stephens, C.N.C

5 HTP. It sometimes stops premenstrual symptoms. Often, I combine it with L-theanine, St. John's Wort, L-tyrosine, or NADH for greater benefit.

Most begin 5 HTP by taking 50 milligrams twice a day. If no improvement occurs, dosages can be increased to 100 milligrams up to two or three times a day. The proper dosage can ensure success.

It is not recommended to combine 5 HTP with a conventional antidepressant without doctor's permission.

L-Theanine

L-Theanine is an amino acid found in green tea. It supports calmness and clarity of thinking. It's associated with better sleep, less anxiety, improved mood, and brain clarity. This supplement rarely lets me down.

An experiment conducted in Shizuoka, Japan, at the Laboratory of Nutritional Biology, found that dopamine concentrations in the brain, especially in the hypothalamus, striatum, and hippocampus, increased significantly after the administration of L-Theanine.[103]

Most start with 100 milligrams of L-Theanine two to three times a day. Some need a higher dosage for optimal effect.

Frank

Recently, a pilot with anxiety problems told me that he could not take anti-anxiety medications and fly. He told me he started taking L-Theanine and found that it worked better for him than any anti-anxiety medication ever did. The L-theanine does not sedate him.

St. John's Wort

St. John's Wort has been used regularly in Europe to treat depression, fibromyalgia, sleep disorders, and viral infections. It makes more serotonin and dopamine available.

Dr. Michael Murray, author of *Encyclopedia for Natural Medicine*, says, "St. John's Wort extract (300 mg., 0.3 hypericin content) can work well in fibromyalgia patients, especially when it is mixed with 5 HTP and magnesium. The combination works better than either alone."[104] The dosage of St. John's Wort is often 300 milligrams three times a day. Do not mix with conventional antidepressants.

L-Tyrosine

The amino acid L-tyrosine is a building block of dopamine and norepinephrine. It is used to enhance mental alertness and relieve depression. I have also seen it improve energy and reduce fibromyalgia pain. I start most clients on 500 to 1,000 milligrams twice a day. It is best to start low and work up. L-tyrosine also supports the thyroid gland. Avoid L-tyrosine if you are taking an MAO-inhibitor drug for depression.

Dosing of Medications and Supplements

One of the most important things I have learned with medications that affect brain chemicals and hormones is that there is a very small therapeutic window where they work well. What this means is if your dosage is too low, likely you will see no improvements; or if too high, you could even feel worse. The surest way to avoid problems and find the just-right dosage is to start low and work up slowly until improvements are noted.

Patricia Stephens, C.N.C

Quality Counts

The positive side of natural supplements is that, after working with them for ten years, I find that quality brands are safe and effective. Inexpensive supplements do not always work. There can be an enormous difference between low-cost supplements versus high-quality supplements.

Even though there is no FDA (Food and Drug Administration) regulation on supplements, there are many companies that produce pharmaceutical-grade supplements, which have enough of the active ingredients to work effectively. Some supplement companies sell their products only to doctors or pharmacists. They guard their reputations carefully. Buying inexpensive supplements is usually not a bargain.

Summary

- Many medical professionals are not currently aware of the link between low dopamine and/ or norepinephrine levels and chronic pain or other chronic symptoms. Perhaps part of the reason for this is mainstream medicine has generally focused more on imbalances in serotonin. (Some of the newer medications enhance the work of serotonin and norepinephrine.) Many of the medications used to improve dopamine and norepinephrine have basically not been used for any conditions other than AD/HD and narcolepsy. Because most of the AD/HD medications have been used mainly in children, it would be likely to miss the connection between other symptoms of low dopamine and norepinephrine, such as chronic pain, that would usually show up later in life. However, now good medical documentation is surfacing that demonstrates this connection.

- Hormones and neurotransmitters work interactively.

- Increasing dopamine and other supportive brain chemicals can improve energy, mood, memory, sleep, and lessen or eliminate pain.

- I always try to screen FMS and other chronically ill clients for hormonal imbalances. Hormonal imbalances can be at the root of many chronic symptoms. Hormones can help the body make more brain chemicals like serotonin, dopamine and norepinephrine.

- Dosage is critical for medications and supplements which affect dopamine. If the dosage is too low, benefit will not result. If the levels are too high, you can feel worse. The best way to avoid the problem is to start low and work up. There can be a small therapeutic window where one feels best.

- Although the first one usually works, some supplements and medications which affect dopamine might be more effective for you than others. A good analogy for this is that they are like keys that fit a lock. The right key is the one that opens the door for you.

- Sometimes, combining supplements delivers the best results.

Serotonin: A Feel-Good Brain Chemical

An important neurotransmitter that improves overall well-being is serotonin. When it is low or out of balance, various symptoms can occur.

Establishing a Connection between Depression and Pain

Scientists have long noted benefits from medications that affect serotonin, such as balanced mood, sleep, and energy. These medications have also been used in patients with migraine headaches, eating disorders, depression, obesity, PMS, anxiety disorder, panic attacks, alcoholism, and fibromyalgia. Sometimes these medications control symptoms, and other times they do not.

Many physicians believe there is a connection between pain and depression. According to Daniel Hall-Flavin, MD, psychiatrist at Mayo Clinic,

> Doctors who treat chronic pain and depression have known for many years how closely these two

conditions are linked. Some research shows that pain and depression share common pathways in the emotional (limbic) region of the brain. Certain antidepressants may relieve pain in some people by reducing their pain perception.[105]

If you desire to use supplements, with or without prescription medications, make your doctor aware. Usually supplements mix well with medications, but interactions might rarely happen. Proceed with caution.

Serotonin Plays Many Roles

Studies also link serotonin to pain perception, headaches, and mood disorders. Regina P. Gilliland, MD, an Internist at the Mobile Infirmary Medical Center, states, "The most widely acknowledged biochemical abnormality associated with fibromyalgia is low serotonin levels."[106] Note the "most widely acknowledged biochemical abnormality" means what is mainly endorsed by the medical community to date.

Serotonin and other neurotransmitters have a profound effect on overall health and well-being. Correcting chemical imbalances can improve symptoms which may accompany depression.

Balancing Serotonin with Norepinephrine and Dopamine

There are many cases of "refractory" depression, which is depression that doesn't respond to standard treatment. Many doctors use treatment programs that focus on serotonin, but some doctors are combining medications for greater benefit. Currently, there is a newer class of medications called serotonin and norepinephrine reuptake inhibitors (SNRIs), and sometimes patients will respond to them when they have not responded positively to medications that affect only serotonin.

If you are taking a medication currently that affects mainly serotonin, and you have not found the relief you are looking for, consider asking your doctor about addressing imbalances in two other brain chemicals, dopamine and norepinephrine. Also, consider correcting hormonal imbalances.

Coming Face to Face with
My Own Depression

Years ago, after visiting too many doctors for various physical complaints, one of my doctors told me I was depressed. For some reason, that made me furious. I did not have the symptoms of depression, in my mind's eye, such as the blues, crying spells, and irritability. Instead, what I did have was pain and plenty of it.

Eventually, I did try some antidepressants, which did not decrease the pain or make me feel better. In my mind, that meant that I really was not depressed. What I did not know at the time is I had not used the right combination of medications.

Finally, after having a SPECT Scan, which showed a lack of blood flowing into some regions of my brain, a symptom usually seen in depressed patients, I began to accept the diagnosis of depression. At this point, I became actively involved in finding the right treatment regimen.

My Perspective

Years ago, when I took medications that affected just serotonin, such as SSRIs (antidepressants which are selective serotonin reuptake inhibitors), I saw no basic improvement. Later, when I took a stimulant medication (which affects dopamine and norepinephrine), I had mixed results, until I added back a low-dose serotonin medication to it to stabilize my chemistry. The combination stopped my uneven response. As a post-menopausal woman, I was also on estrogen at the time, which was also a critical part of my regimen. This combination dramatically improved my quality of life.

> When I combined a stimulant and an anti-depressant, all FMS symptoms went away, including all the pain.

Restoring Brain Chemical Balance:
The Journey to Reward

All of these medications and supplements are like keys to a lock. Some medications and supplements that affect missing brain chemicals work better for some individuals than others. For me, even though bupropion relieved my pain, I later found that stimulants used to treat AD/HD worked better. It all boils down to trial and error. For some it comes easy; others find it takes some real work.

I wrestled for months, attempting to bring balance to my brain chemistry with various medications affecting different brain chemicals. At this time, nothing was in print regarding an FMS and AD/HD connection. I found myself in uncharted waters.

> The following thoughts kept me moving when I wanted to quit: The doctors have said you will have to live with your diagnosis. There is no cure. I then had to ask myself these questions: Can I accept this? Do I believe this? What have they missed? Can I be a part of reversing my own prognosis? How hard am I willing to work to find relief from this misery? The rest is history. The win was worth the work.

Natural Alternatives to Balance Serotonin

There are some wonderful supplements that work well to balance serotonin. I have observed benefit too many times to doubt their effectiveness. They are excellent, generally, for mild to moderate depression. Others will need something stronger, like a prescription.

Some supplements might work better for your chemistry than others. SAM-e is generally considered the most potent. However, it is usually much more expensive.

You can easily locate more information on the Internet regarding supplements, which include dosages and safety. I encourage you to do your own research. That is how I have brought this information to you.

Remember that the following supplements not only affect serotonin, but often enhance other brain chemicals. Because of this, there will be some repetition from the earlier chapters.

5-Hydroxytryptophan (5-HTP)

Most begin with 50 milligrams twice daily. If no benefit after a week, doses are often increased to 100 milligrams two to three times daily. Most notice improvements within two weeks, but not all. It can take four or more weeks to experience full therapeutic effect.

I have seen very impressive improvements in clients suffering from depression, stress, anxiety, and fibromyalgia while using 5 HTP.

St. John's Wort

Most find 300 milligrams two to three times a day sufficient. Some take 600 milligrams at a time. The product should contain 0.3 percent hypericin, the most commonly studied active ingredient.

St. John's Wort and 5 HTP both have been reported to help improve sleep when the dosage is therapeutic. It often works alone, but it can work better when combined with other supplements. A high quality product works best.

SAM-e

Most begin with 200 milligrams twice daily on an *empty stomach.* In a week, if there is no improvement, most go up to 400 milligrams twice daily. Some use even more. Once improvements are noted, many can decrease to a maintenance dosage of 200 milligrams twice daily. A few have some gastrointestinal discomfort, which may be related to too high of a dosage. This will usually go away.

SAM-e has been reported to assist liver health, reduce or stop aches and pains, and improve mood. Some sources report improvements in mood within a week. *Pain relief can take five to six weeks.*

Even though SAM-e is a more expensive choice, I have seen it work when other supplements failed. However, I usually suggest that my clients try the less expensive products first.

Do not take SAM-e if you have been diagnosed with bi-polar/manic depression without your doctor's approval.

Inositol

In double-blind trials, twelve to eighteen grams of Inositol per day has shown to be effective for depression, anxiety and obsessive compulsive disorder.[107] Because of individual dosing needs, some might need less.

Inositol is a member of B Complex, which helps in serotonin activity modulation. Neurotransmitters in the brain depend on Inositol to function properly. "Low levels of this nutrient may result in depression and some research has shown that increased levels of Inositol appear to be a promising treatment of depression." [108] In fact, in a double-blind controlled trial using twelve grams of Inositol daily showed "significant overall benefit for (those using) Inositol compared to placebo (sugar pill) was found at week four on the Hamilton Depression Scale. (Smaller dosages are better initially.) Inositol significantly reduced scores of obsessive compulsive disorder compared with placebo."[109]

B Complex

Many find that a good B Complex improves energy, brain function, and mood.

B vitamins are supportive in the production of many brain chemicals. I put most of my clients with hormonal or suspected brain chemical imbalances on a good B complex. Most notice improved energy and well-being.

Do not take 5 HTP, St. John's Wort, or SAM-e with conventional antidepressant without first discussing it with your doctor. Correct dosing can be critical to success.

Side Effects of Supplements

After taking supplements and seeing their effects on others, I must say that natural supplements can cause side effects. When side effects occur, they are generally mild and go away in a day or two after stopping the supplement. Generally, the degree of side effect is nothing like I have experienced with conventional psychotropic (mind-altering) medications. After consulting with clients using supplements, I have never seen any long-lasting side effects after discontinuing supplements.

> When I have a problem with a medication or supplement, I *usually* find the problem will go away when the dosage is *decreased*, or it will go away over time as my body adjusts to it.

A Note For Sensitive Patients

Because some fibromyalgia and other chronically ill patients are extremely sensitive, I always recommend starting my sensitive clients on one quarter to one half the recommended dosages. Then, they can work up slowly. A small dosage often works as effectively for them as a large dosage for others.

I am very sensitive personally. When I experience a slight negative response, as long as it is not too significant, I keep taking it a few days. Often, a negative reaction will go away in a few days to a week as the body adjusts to it.

Summary

• Serotonin is an extremely important neurotransmitter. When it is low, significant symptoms can develop, such as depression, mood swings, cognitive problems, sleep disturbances, headaches, other various aches and pains, low energy, weight gain or weight loss and food cravings. Low levels have been documented widely in FMS and other chronically ill patients. Improving serotonin alone seems to help only marginally in most FMS and other chronically ill patients that I have come in contact with.

- Serotonin is just one of the three brain chemicals that can really reverse many of the symptoms of chronic disease discussed in this book. Remember, not only serotonin needs to be balanced. I believe balancing dopamine, norepinephrine, and serotonin will have the most profound effect on fibromyalgia and possibly other chronic disease states.

- Dosage can be critical to success, whether using conventional medications or natural supplements. A few need small dosages, and others need much more to benefit.

- Remember, there are also safe and effective natural alternatives to balance serotonin for mild to moderate depression. The most commonly used supplements are 5 HTP, St. John's Wort, and SAM-e. *These should not be mixed with conventional antidepressant medications unless under the supervision of a physician.*

Digestive Health

Many chronically-ill people frequently experience gastrointestinal disturbances. Making improvements in the gastrointestinal system can improve overall health and well-being.

Unless we are digesting foods thoroughly, absorbing the nutrients, and ridding our bodies of the waste material, chronic health concerns can surface.

Fortunately, alternative therapies have been successfully used to correct gastrointestinal imbalances. I have seen the therapies described in this chapter make a significant difference.

The main focus of this book is not gastrointestinal health, but improving digestive health can improve a large array of symptoms, including those of hormonal imbalance.

The Brain/Gut Connection

Ever feel nauseated when someone upsets you or when you did something you regretted? Nearly everyone has, but few of us consciously make the connection between the nervous and digestive systems.

Interestingly, neurotransmitters, such as serotonin, are not only in the brain but are also made in the gastrointestinal system. These neurotransmitters enhance communication between nerve cells, muscles, and glands. According to Michael Gershon, MD, in his book, *The Second Brain*, "every class of neurotransmitter found in the brain is also found in the enteric nervous system,"[110] which is a highly integrated nervous system within the wall of the intestine.[111]

The lining of the small intestinal mucosa is highly specialized for maximizing digestion and absorption of nutrients. The lining also produces chemicals, which help digestion and improve immune defenses, and hormones that coordinate digestive processes of the intestine, gallbladder, and pancreas.[112]

The entire body is interconnected, and a healthy, optimally functioning gastrointestinal system is critical to good health. But finding cause and effect gets extremely complicated.

The Challenges of Digestion

The twenty-first century lifestyle discourages optimal digestion because we are eating on the run and are under stress while eating. Many of us have forgotten how to truly relax. Our minds and bodies are continually racing. Maybe we don't even sit down with our families to an uninterrupted, healthy meal. Considerable amounts of our food contain unnatural ingredients that our bodies find difficult to digest. Additionally, highly processed foods usually lack nutrients our bodies need to properly function.

Just a few of these unnatural substances that we are consuming are preservatives, pesticides sprayed on

Patricia Stephens, C.N.C

fruits and vegetables, and chlorinated water. Our bodies also come in contact with pollutants and toxins that need to be metabolized and excreted. If not, they are stored in body tissues where they can cause problems not often linked to the source.

Another challenge is that, as we age, our digestion slows down. This affects how we break down and use the nutrients in our foods.

Also overcooking vegetables and storing foods too long (either at home or through shipment) can affect nutritional content.

Brenda Watson, founder of Renew Life, a leading company whose focus is restoring gastrointestinal health, is a respected author and speaker. She has formulated some effective products that help treat or reverse chronic gastrointestinal problems. She states in her book, *Renew Your Life*, "It is estimated that as much as 40% of the population suffer from some form of digestive stress."[113]

As you see, gastrointestinal problems are very common. The following information is an introduction to alternative therapies used to improve gastrointestinal health and correct gastrointestinal complaints.

Correcting the Digestive Dilemma

Jeffery Bland, Chief Science Officer of Metagenics, in his Health Comm publication called "The Four R's," provides a tool that is highly regarded by many alternative practioners for assessing chronic complaints.[114] These steps can transform health.

Rule One: Remove

Alternative practioners usually consider problem foods, or IgG food sensitivities, as major contributors to chronic illness. As an example, for those sensitive to gluten, a protein found in many grains, removing gluten from the diet can quickly provide symptomatic relief. Common offending foods are milk, wheat, corn, egg whites, soy, and peanuts. Not everyone with chronic health concerns is sensitive to all these, but food sensitivities can significantly compromise health.

Removing foods which produce dysbiosis, an overgrowth of the unhealthy organisms in the colon, can help restore health to the gastrointestinal system and the body.

Removing sugar from the diet, in some, can stop pain completely and quickly. I have seen this many times. Removing sugar can improve many other complaints. Some are sensitive to it and others are not.

These offending foods are not usually found on popular IgE-food-allergy tests, but often will show up on IgG-food-sensitivity tests. IgE food allergies result in an *immediate* response such as swelling of lips, face, and eyes or difficulty breathing. IgG food sensitivities are foods that induce a *delayed* response, from two hours to four days after ingesting.

Many conventional doctors do not consider IgG food sensitivities as important, but most naturopathic professionals believe removing IgG food sensitivities to be extremely important in reversing chronic disease. I have seen significant improvements personally and in others after removing IgG food sensitivities.

IgG-related symptoms can vary widely. Just a few symptoms are migraine headaches, aches and pains,

_____ *Patricia Stephens, C.N.C*

gastrointestinal problems, low energy, high blood pressure, and weight gain. James Braly, MD, states,

> Delayed food reactions can emanate (come from) from any organ or tissue in the human body, provoking over 100 allergic symptoms and well over 150 different medical diseases. An estimated 60 to 80 million Americans suffer from clinically significant food allergies, most all of whom suffer delayed symptoms.[115]

I usually encourage my chronically-ill clients to stop consuming dairy products completely because it is a common, significant offender for those with chronic health problems. Often lactose is not the only problem. Casein, a protein in dairy products, can cause significant problems. If you are concerned about getting calcium, it can be replaced by consuming other calcium rich foods, or by supplementation. There are excellent milk replacements such as rice, almond, oat, and soy milk. They are readily available in most grocery stores and are pleasant tasting. If removing dairy products does not help, then other common allergens can be removed through guesswork or testing. *A small amount of a sensitive food can cause a big problem.*

Try completely removing a suspicious food for two to three weeks to see if symptoms improve. Afterward, the food can be reintroduced to see if symptoms return. If you return a food to your diet that you are sensitive to, the response is usually powerful. It may occur immediately, or it may take up to four days. If you do not feel worse after reintroducing the food, the food should be fine.

IgG sensitivities can be tested by many labs throughout the country. This can remove the guesswork. Some of the reputable labs are:

- Metametrix,
  http://www.metametrix.com/content/Home
- US Biotek, http://www.usbiotek.com
- Genova Diagnosics http://www.gdx.net/home
- Better Health USA,
  http://www.betterhealthusa.
  com/public/282.cfm

Removing yeast overgrowth and other pathogens, such as bacteria or viruses, can also be very helpful for many patients. Many alternative practitioners address candida overgrowth in chronically-ill patients. Factors contributing to yeast overgrowth include repeated antibiotic therapy, compromised immune systems, too much dietary sugar, stress, hormonal imbalances, medications such as steroids, and birth control pills.

Supplements can assist in removal of yeast overgrowth. Some are combination products formulated to rid the body of excess yeast. Other effective supplements are olive leaf extract, garlic, oil of oregano, caprylic acid, and grapefruit seed extract. High potency probiotics can also be beneficial. Chronically-ill patients should remove yeast slowly. Some patients experience a negative response. I recommend my clients start low and work up on the dosages. Do more research on the Herxheimer Response or healing crisis so you are better informed. Candida questionnaires can be found online.

Patricia Stephens, C.N.C

Rule Two: Replace Enzymes
I have seen impressive benefits when using digestive enzymes. They help fight inflammation, improve digestion, help solve hormone-related sympton, and can improve the absorption of all nutrients in foods as well as supplements.

Ned

A man suffering from significant heartburn was seeking relief. His sleep was interrupted, and he had a lot of esophageal pain. I recommended a high-powered digestive enzyme and told him to take two of them with a meal. He came by in a few weeks to tell me that, since the first day of taking these enzymes with each meal, he had not had heartburn. His words were, "It is a miracle!"

> Never underestimate the power of digestive enzymes.

Many professionals tell us that as we age, we have too much stomach acid, when in reality, large numbers of those over forty often have insufficient levels of stomach acid. Stomach acid must be present to break down proteins and minerals and kill bacteria in our foods. When our foods are not being digested and just sit in our stomachs or intestines, they can ferment or rot. *Rotting food gives off acids.* Effectively moving foods through the digestive system usually stops the acid-producing fermentation.

Digestive enzymes can be purchased with or without hydrochloric acid (HCl). Many are low in hydrochloric acid and others are not. Getting the right enzyme product can be helpful, especially in the aging adult.

This is a test you can use to assess whether your levels of stomach acid are low or high. Mix one tablespoon of apple cider vinegar with eight ounces of water and drink with a meal. If pain or warmth is felt soon thereafter in the stomach, this is a sign that HCI is sufficient. If no problem or benefit is noted, take two tablespoons with a meal to assess if there is any warmth or pain. If no warmth or pain is noted, continue to add one tablespoon at each meal until a warm sensation in the stomach is experienced, then decrease the amount of vinegar by one tablespoon.[116] In other words, dosing is very important. Some use one to two teaspoons with good results. If you experience burning, an antacid will check this discomfort until it goes away. If there is no burning, you probably do not have over-production of acid and might benefit from supplementation.

Rule Three: Reinoculate (replenish):
A healthy intestine has five to seven pounds of healthy bacteria, which are responsible for making vitamins and other resources needed for bodily functioning. A diseased intestine has an imbalance of these bacteria, or a deficiency of the friendly bacteria. These good bacteria are often replaced with pathogenic organisms, which can include yeast overgrowth. You can reinoculate, or replenish, these by taking probiotics, which are healthy strains of good bacteria such as lactobacillus acidophilus, bifidobacterium, and bulgaricus. Also, some foods such as organic yogurt, miso, kefir, and fermented foods, such as sauerkraut and kimchi, are rich in naturally occurring probiotics.

_____ *Patricia Stephens, C.N.C*

We are currently seeing a lot of media attention devoted to probiotics, which are found in yogurt and other fermented foods, but the use of probiotics is not new. Dr. Elias Metchnikoff, a Nobel Prize winner in the early 1900s, was a staunch supporter of using friendly bacteria (probiotics) to improve health and reverse health problems. He considered gastrointestinal health as primary to good health. One of his popular quotes is, "Death begins in the colon."

Brenda Watson, ND (naturopathic doctor), and Leonard Smith, MD, state in their book *Gut Solutions*, "Restoring the optimal bacterial balance in the GI tract is vital to full recovery of health." Beneficial bacteria in the GI tract serve many vital functions. They produce certain B vitamins and also control growth of harmful bacteria, break down toxins, and stimulate the immune system.[117]

Rule Four: Repair

The lining in the small intestine can become unhealthy or even permeable. Once compromised, this formerly protective layer may now allow antigens, something foreign to the body, to evoke an immune response. It also allows other incomplete digestive products to pass through the bowel wall.

Nutrients like L-glutamine, B vitamins, zinc, and vitamin C can improve integrity of the intestinal wall. The job is more easily done when food sensitivities are temporarily removed, anti-inflammatory supplements are used, probiotics are incorporated, healthy foods replace an unhealthy diet, and digestive enzymes are taken with meals.

Some supplements used to reduce inflammation in the colon are curcumin, bromelain, quercetin, ginger, and enteric-coated fish oils. When you slow down inflammation, the body can heal faster.

Constipation

Many chronically-ill patients are chronically constipated. The following suggestions should help alleviate chronic constipation.

1. Increased intake of purified water. A guide is to divide your weight by two. This is the number of ounces of water you need per day.
2. Probiotics
3. Magnesium (dosage matters)
4. Vitamin C (dosage matters)
5. Liver cleansing
6. Omega oils
7. Fiber
8. Cape Aloe
9. Sorbitol
10. Herbal products with sena and cascara (It is best to use these only occasionally.)
11. Exercise

Herbal cleanses and colonics have also been helpful in chronic constipation cases.

For those unfamiliar with colon therapy or colonics, it is a gentle and effective cleansing and stimulation of the large intestine. It is useful in the treatment of digestive disorders and should be accompanied by supportive nutritional guidance. See www.i-act.org .

Diarrhea

Probiotics and fiber have worked well in my clients to reverse chronic diarrhea. Because these clients are often low in minerals, they feel much better incorporating vitamins and minerals in their supplement regimen.

Crohn's disease and colitis need additional support.

Detoxification

Clearing toxins can dramatically improve health. I have found nutritional response testing to be very helpful. It can be used to carefully reduce the toxic load in the body, which can foster impressive improvements. www.unsinc.info/

Summary

- It is impossible to separate good health from gastrointestinal health. The steps of restoring gastrointestinal health are:

  1. Removing problem foods

  2. Ridding the body of candida overgrowth

  3. Restoring nutrition

  4. Improving digestion with digestive enzymes, which often help to lessen pain

  5. Replacing good bacteria in the colon with probiotics

  6. Restoring health to the gut lining, which is your body's first line of immune defense by using supplements such as L-glutamine

- The digestive system is much like the roots of a tree. If the tree has diseased roots, the whole tree is affected. Nutrition, digestion, bacterial balance, absorption, and intestinal permeability all have interdependent functions in the health of the gastrointestinal tract, which affects the health of the entire body.

- Alternative therapies provide relief to patients with chronic gastrointestinal problems over time.

I have seen very impressive changes when these corrections have been made.

Lifestyle Changes that Influence Health

Many of my clients want me to give them a pill that fixes everything without changing their lifestyles or diets. If I do suggest a supplement, some complain about the size or taste of pills, and many don't want to take pills more than once a day—and then only if they think of it. These people have no passion to get well. Their lack of discipline can be a barrier to recovery using natural therapies.

The main goal for many people is symptomatic relief, leaving their lifestyle and diet as is. The information outlined in this book will provide some symptomatic relief even if the diet is not changed. However, when patients are looking for the *roots* of chronic disease, correcting the diet can be a very important part in improving health.

If you are serious about restoring your health and willing to work to get well, this chapter is for you. It contains the lifestyle changes needed to assist you on your journey. This is the "work" chapter. So, are you sick and tired enough to roll up your sleeves and go to work?

Diet

Dietary changes are probably one of our hardest challenges. Food is comforting, and most of us seek some form of comfort in the foods we eat. The thought of eliminating favorite foods or learning to like new foods seems almost overwhelming.

Many people I talk to work and meet the needs of their family, but do not feel healthy. Diet, stress, and lack of rest are usually contributing factors.

Guidelines for Healthy Eating

Healthy eating consists of consuming healthy fats, fewer processed and junk foods, more fresh fruits and vegetables, good lean meats, and whole grains.

Fruits and Vegetables

Fruits and vegetables are packed with vitamins, minerals, and fiber. They are rich in nutrients that improve health at many levels.

The American Cancer Society recommends eating five or more servings of fruits and vegetables daily to help prevent cancer. These foods contain important vitamins, minerals, phytochemicals, and antioxidants and are usually low in calories. In general, those with the most color—green, red, yellow, and orange—have the most nutrients.[118]

Fresh fruits and vegetables not only fight cancer, but they provide nutrients to fight a wide array of other diseases.

Vegetables need to be carefully cooked so they maintain their nutrients. Stir frying, roasting, and steaming are excellent ways to prepare them for optimal nutrition. Roasting is one of my favorite ways to cook vegetables because it brings out their natural sweetness.

Patricia Stephens, C.N.C

To roast vegetables, preheat the oven to 425 degr. Cut up various vegetables into small, fairly unifoı sized cubes. Vegetables like yellow squash, zucchini, reı peppers, red onions, and eggplant work well. However, you can roast most vegetables. Stirring in a handful of fresh herbs like oregano, basil, and thyme from the garden adds flavor. Pour in a small amount of olive oil to lightly coat vegetables. Put vegetables in a low-sided pan. Roast about thirty to forty minutes, or until some vegetables tips are brown. After removing from the oven, sprinkle with sea salt and fresh parmesan cheese.

Lean Meats

Good choices are lean meats, such as chicken, turkey, and fish. Instead of frying, it is best to bake, broil, or pan-fry in olive oil. Be sure to include protein-rich foods with each meal. Good plant sources of protein are some beans and peas. Protein supports blood sugar balance and many other important functions in the body.

Healthy, Whole Grains

Whole grains are generally unprocessed or unrefined. They are excellent sources of fiber. All types of whole grains are excellent sources of complex carbohydrates, vitamins, and minerals, like potassium, magnesium, and selenium.[119] Whole grains provide nutrients that are often low in the standard American diet. You will feel full longer after eating whole grains versus processed grains.

Healthy Fats

Olive oil is a monounsaturated fat that is excellent for cooking and baking. Also, butter is an excellent choice in cooking and baking in moderation.

Other types of fats can cause health problems, but do not

Statistics show that nearly 99 percent of people in the United States do not eat enough omega 3 fatty acids. The symptoms of omega 3 fatty acid deficiency can be very vague and can often be labeled as some other health condition.

Snack Foods
Most of us love the wrong kinds of snacks. It takes conscious effort to incorporate healthy ones into our diet. When possible, consume snacks such as small amounts of nuts or nut butters, fresh fruit, whole-wheat crackers, carrots, celery sticks, or protein bars. Junk foods like potato chips are usually expensive, high fat, and nutritionally empty.

Foods to Avoid or Reduce

1. Simple carbohydrates, including large amounts of sugar. Instead, stick with complex carbohydrates like whole grains.

2. High fat foods and snacks.

3. Cow's milk- Not all, but many with chronic health problems have problems digesting cow's milk. Remove to see if you feel better after avoiding it for two to three weeks. If not, most put it back in their diet, if desired.

4. Other foods you are sensitive to. (The most common food sensitivities are dairy, wheat, corn, and eggs. However, you can be sensitive to any food. These foods can cause significant problems. Further described in "Digestive Health" chapter.)

Healthy Sweeteners

Most of us love something sweet to eat. Including moderate amounts of natural sweeteners like honey, xylitol, stevia, agave, molasses, maple syrup, and lo han can be better ways to satisfy your sweet tooth. If you are having sugar cravings, there are good supplements that will help reduce them like hoodia, gymnema sylvestre, and L-glutamine.

A Realistic Dietary Plan

Perhaps this is an area where you need to make changes. Try to create a realistic plan, one you can follow over the long term. If you change your diet too drastically, you may not be able to stay with it. It might be easier for you to make long-term changes if you reduce some of the unhealthy foods in your diet before stopping them completely.

One thing I have learned is I am capable of changing my diet. After I begin to feel better and adjust to eating new foods, sticking with the changes becomes easier. I don't eat perfectly, but generally I consume a healthy diet. Once you feel better, you may be able to cheat a little more and still feel well.

Nutritional Deficiencies

Many people think they are eating healthy, when, in reality, many are not. Despite living in a land of plenty, they may be in a state of nutritional deficiency.

A key problem is low levels of various vitamins and minerals. Many clients feel better after adding a high-quality whole foods multivitamin. Seeing their improvements tells me they were not getting enough nutrients from their diet. Most tell me they see improvements

Patricia Stephens, C.N.C

like more energy, better brain performance and stronger immunity.

Remember, if our digestion is poor, we may not be breaking down foods properly to absorb nutrients.

Stress Reduction

Our stressful lives are counterproductive to good health because stress places ever-increasing demands on us. Our bodies have been designed to do repair work when they have rest, proper nutrition, and adequate hormones and brain chemicals to keep bodily functions running smoothly.

Ways to Reduce Stress

1. Slow down. Learn to relax.

2. Don't overload your schedule.

3. Be realistic. Don't expect so much of yourself.

4. Get enough rest.

5. Delegate jobs to others who are capable.

6. De-clutter your life and keep things as simple as possible.

7. Pace yourself so you are less exhausted at the end of the day.

8. Focus on the best in other people.

9. Take one day at a time.

10. Live within your means.

11. Do something for pleasure each day. You may have to put this on the calendar.

12. Allow yourself extra time so you are less rushed. Set the clock earlier.

13. Eat healthy foods. Sharply reduce junk foods.

14. Find a way to improve your organizational system.

15. Every day, find time to be alone so you can dream.

16. Laugh, laugh and laugh some more. Watch comedies, or spend time with a friend with a sense of humor.

17. Get a day-planner.

18. Take yourself less seriously.

19. Forgive others.

20. Count your blessings.

The Art of Making Good Choices

A beginning place is to prioritize how we spend resources of energy, time, and money to improve the quality of our lives. We need to be careful not to trade long-term health for short-term wealth. Perhaps we have unconsciously equated busyness with productivity. Most of us take little time to plan, dream, relax, and reflect. Learning to separate the urgent from the important is a daily task for each of us. Most of us spend too much time making a living instead of making a life.

Because women are caregivers by nature, we can spend all our energies caring for others and neglecting ourselves. We need to learn to delegate and set aside a little time, even if it is a few minutes each day, to do something pleasurable.

At times, you may feel circumstances are out of your control. The reality is, we all have choices. We hold some of the controls. We can prioritize, make changes,

_____ *Patricia Stephens, C.N.C*

and eliminate what's really not that important. We can weigh everything against the bigger picture.

Trust me on this one. Health is fragile. *It is easier to nourish good health than to recover from chronic disease.* A balanced life is a critical element for quality living.

Sleep

Getting enough sleep is very important to good health, but many of us can't seem to turn our minds off in order to relax at bedtime. Improving nighttime conditions will usually improve sleep quality. Because watching TV and working on the computer can be highly stimulating, turning these off one to two hours before bedtime can be helpful. Other good ideas can be making the temperature of the room comfortable, getting the room as dark as possible, having a light snack including a little protein before bed, and meditating before bed.

Some, after doing all of the above, still need a supplement or a medication to support sleep. Magnesium, L-theanine, 5 HTP, valerian are just some of the supplements that support restful sleep. Others need something stronger to make their bodies rest.

Balancing hormones and brain chemicals can help the body sleep more naturally without medications, or at least that is what I have seen in myself and a lot of other clients.

Exercise

Doctors tell chronically-ill patients to get exercise, which is good advice. The problem is, when you're sick, you may not have energy to exercise, at least not initially. When you start, exercise slowly and build up over time. Eventually you should notice more energy.

You can start with effective, low-impact exercise, such as walking and water exercise.

Years ago, when my doctors told me to get exercise, I remember thinking they had no clue how low my energy was. Their command seemed like "mission impossible" to me. However, I began to walk short distances, and, over time, my stamina increased.

In the beginning, it took all the energy I had to cross the room. Today, I can exercise moderately for an hour without feeling any recurrence of symptoms. Getting my brain chemistry and hormones balanced has made a big difference in my stamina and energy.

Summary

- Incorporating lifestyle changes into your daily schedule can improve your quality of life. Four goals to strive for are improving diet, reducing stress, improving sleep, and increasing exercise as tolerated.

- Improving your diet will usually correct nutritional deficiencies. Sometimes, a multivitamin is needed to restore levels. Learn to like new foods. Think about what you are eating and how it affects your health. Include more fruits and vegetables, lean meats and whole grains. You can learn to really like these foods, even if they aren't in your current diet.

- Don't underestimate your body's powerful "in-house pharmacy" that is ready to make what is needed to restore and repair your body when it has the right raw materials to do its job. Your efforts will be rewarded with improved health over time.

- Stress can cause many imbalances in the body, which robs overall quality of life. You can make choices regarding how you spend your resources of time, money, and energy. Plan well so you can reduce stress and improve your health and sense of well-being. Learn to say, "No," when you need a break.

- Most of these lifestyle changes are within your reach. You have to decide if you are willing to do the planning and work. I tell my clients, "You are my partner. You are the expert of the body you live in. No one is more interested in your health than you."

- Years ago, I would have thought my recovery was impossible because I was so sick. Yet, I have seen personally how far the body can recover when it has what it needs to do its repair work. I have seen a health miracle, and I believe something better is waiting with your name on it.

- In other words, you can be an active part of your own health miracle.

Summing It Up

This book covers a lot of information. The following list of supplements is basically where I begin with my FMS clients, and many others with chronic health problems. Supplements often work well, but some find that a conventional drug can be stronger and more effective, or at least initially. The benefits of pharmaceutical drugs can be impressive, but sometimes they are heavy laden with side effects. (I have not seen that with stimulants *when the dosage is correct*.) What matters most is what works better for you with the least side effects or problems.

Remember, it may take time and effort to find what works best for your body. Step up to become your own advocate. No one is more interested in your health than you are.

Alternative Options

If you decide to pursue natural alternatives, consider trying the following supplements. (More detailed information is included in the previous chapters.) There are many other very effective supplements, but the following can provide a good starting place to improve FMS and other chronic problems.

Improving Brain Chemical Balance
(From the following choices, I begin with one to see how the client responds. Before we add anything new, we work with the dosage to make sure they are taking enough. If they still are not feeling optimal, I often add something else for greater effectiveness.)

1. 5 HTP- I start my clients on one 50-milligram capsule twice a day for a week. If no change, we go up to two twice a week. Sometimes this supplement works quickly, and other times it takes two weeks to show improvements. *Do not combine 5 HTP with conventional antidepressants unless your doctor approves.* I have seen it lesson or stop pain, including headaches, improve mood, energy, and sleep.

2. St. John's Wort- It can be used alone or with 5 HTP to support mood and reduce aches and pain. Most start with 300 milligrams twice a day. Some use 300 milligrams three times a day.

3. L-theanine-This supplement is used to stop or lessen anxiety and supports calm focus. It can improve sleep in many. Most start with one to two 100-milligram capsules or tablets two to three times a day. This supplement generally mixes well with conventional medications.

Patricia Stephens, C.N.C

4. SAM-e- Most start SAM-e at 200 milligrams twice a day for a week on an empty stomach. Generally, they see mood benefits in one week. If they are not noticing benefits, they usually elevate the dosage to 400 milligrams twice a day. As they begin to feel better, most, but not all, can lower the dosage to 200 milligrams twice a day. SAM-e has shown impressive changes with aches and pains in about five or six weeks. It can be taken alone or with other supplements like NADH or L-tyrosine. (If SAM-e was not expensive, it would be my first choice, but most do well with 5 HTP or St. John's Wort.) Do not mix SAM-e with conventional antidepressants unless your doctor approves. Do not take with manic depression unless approved by your doctor.

Improving Hormone Balance

Many chronically-ill patients have hormonal imbalances, and correcting them can have a profound effect on their health and quality of life. After assessing levels through saliva of most women with chronic problems, I find most of them are low in progesterone. I see very impressive benefits when progesterone levels improve at any age. Some are also low in estrogen, but not all. Progesterone, in the natural form, can support relaxation and sleep, reduce aches and pains, and improve mood. I cannot overstress the improvements I have seen when the dosage is and remains correct. Follow-up testing is often advised three months after beginning supplementation or hormonal replacement therapy to make sure balance has been achieved. It is fairly inexpensive to retest because only the hormones that were out of balance are re-tested.

After balancing estrogen, progesterone, and testosterone, if symptoms remain, or if it is difficult to balance female or male hormones, consider imbalances that might be present in the adrenal or thyroid gland. Correcting imbalances in thyroid and adrenal hormones can make a profound difference in health and quality of life.

Other Important Factors to Consider are:

1. Ridding the Body of Toxins
2. Improving Gastrointestinal Health
3. Improving Diet and Lifestyle
4. Correcting Mineral Deficiencies–Magnesium can help chronic complaints.

Supplements can be initially added to control pain. Some good choices are hyaluronic acid, MSM, curcumin, boswellia, or malic acid.

Conventional Options

Because many of you need treatment options covered under insurance, or trust only what is prescribed by a doctor, I have included information on some prescription medications. Even though this was the first way I found much needed dramatic relief, it is not my first choice currently. My heart is in helping people find what is out of balance in their bodies and correcting these imbalances. However, because I have seen these medications stop long-standing pains and improve other symptoms as early as the first day they were used, I must include this information.

Many medications covered in this book are not part of mainstream medicine's treatment for chronic pain and other chronic problems. Because of this, I believe conventional medicine needs to take a good look at this. Too many people are suffering with debilitating pain and other symptoms that rob our quality of life.

Another reason I endorse this is because some people do not readily embrace programs requiring a lot of work. Others do not want to change their diets to feel better. They want something to take care of the symptoms, and they can live with the rest. If this is you, conventional options might be the best choice.

Wellbutrin

This is a prescription antidepressant that affects the neurotransmitters dopamine and norepinephrine, two of the neurotransmitters that I believe are out of balance in a large number of FMS patients and perhaps other chronic illnesses.

This medication can be called in by your physician. *Many doctors combine it with other antidepressant medications that affect serotonin.* Some do well with Wellbutrin alone, but others find they cannot tolerate it by itself. It works differently when it is combined with other medications. It can take five to six weeks to begin working in some patients. Be patient. When people are anxious, it has been combined with Buspar and other medications that affect serotonin. I have seen it greatly lessen or stop FMS pain. It can also improve energy and many other symptoms.

Cymbalta, Lyrica, and Savella

Cymbalta is an SNRI antidepressant which is approved for FMS. Some do well on it. Lyrica has also been approved to treat fibromyalgia and is used to treat other types of chronic pain. Some get good results with it, but many note intolerable side effects from it. Savella is a newly FDA-approved medication for FMS.

Stimulants Used to Treat AD/HD

If one sees himself in the AD/HD criteria, he might consider being screened by a good medical professional such as a psychiatrist, psychologist, or a family practitioner. Carefully check out the doctor to make sure they treat adult AD/HD before making the appointment. If the clinician diagnoses you or a loved one with AD/HD, know that stimulants are the mainstay medications to treat it. Most of the time, no other class of medications works better to clear the symptoms. In fact, you cannot be treated with stimulant medications unless you meet AD/HD criteria or narcolepsy (falling asleep regularly at inappropriate times).

For me, they completely stopped the FMS pain. Often stimulants work very quickly when the patient has the right amount of the right medication and it is taken at the right time of the day.

If you are diagnosed with AD/HD, be prepared to work with stimulant medications. Usually the first medication works, but sometimes one medication will work better than others. The most important consideration is dosage. Improper dosage is the most common error made in treating AD/HD. A small change *in dosage can make a big difference.*

Buspar

This is a good, non-addictive anti-anxiety medication that affects the brain chemical serotonin. It is often combined with other medication like Wellbutrin. I found great relief at one time with this combination.

Other medications have also been discussed in the previous chapters.

> Because I am not a doctor, I would recommend that you discuss these medications with your pharmacist and doctor. Also, become your own advocate for improved health. Step up to become a partner in restored health. Do not forget that the body is designed to heal.

I believe hormonal and brain chemical imbalances have been significantly overlooked in the chronically ill, and correcting these imbalances can greatly improve our quality of life. I also believe it can save you and the health care system a lot of money. That is what I have seen personally and in many others.

I pray for you daily, and believe each of you who are suffering can overcome or dramatically improve your health. *I really want you to feel better. You can. I am sure of it.*

Bibliography

"About Fibromyalgia." UCLA Center for Neurovisceral Sciences and Women's Health. 2 July 2008 <www.cns.med.ucla.edu/PatientFibro.htm>

"Addison's Disease." National Endocrine and Metabolic Diseases Information Services, a service of The National Institute of Diabetes, Digestive and Kidney Diseases. 13 July 2008 <http://www.endocrine.niddk.nih.gov/pubs/addison/addison.htm>

Alternative Medicine Review. 3:3.(1998) 224.

Amen, Daniel, MD *Healing ADD*, G.P. Putman's Sons, 2001.

Amen, Daniel, MD "The Brain Place." The Amen Clinic.<http://amenclinics.com/bp/articles.php?articleID=10>

"Amino Acids." 25 Aug 2007 <http://www.libertyzone.com/hz-Amino-Acid.html>

"Antidepressants: Medicine for Depression." Updated June 2005. 29 Aug 2007. <http://familydoctor.org/online/famdocen/home/common/mentalhealth/treatment/012.html>

Archer, J.S. "Estrogen and mood changes via CNS activity." *Menopausal Medicine.* 7 (1999): 4–8.

Arpels, J.C. "The female brain hypoestrogenic continuum from the premenstrual syndrome to menopause: A hypothesis and review." *Journal of Reproductive Medicine.* 41 (1996): 633–639.

Braly, James, MD, "IgG ELISA Delayed Food Allergy Testing." 3 Sept. 2007 <http://www.drbralyallergyrelief.com/igg.html>

Caruso I. et. al. "Double-blind study of 5-Hydroxytryptophan versus placebo in treatment of primary fibromyalgia syndrome." *J Int Med Res.* 18 (1990) 201–209.

Company Biography. 27 Jan. 2008 <www.diagnostechs.com/main/htm>

"Diagnosis of AD/HD in Adults." National Resource Center on AD/HD. Updated Sept 2005. 17 Sept 2008. 1–2 < http://www.help4adhd.org/en/treatment>

"Fibromyalgia Causes." Mayo Clinic. Updated 4 Oct 2006. 26 Feb 2007, <www.mayoclinic.com/health/fibromyalgia/DS00079/DSECTION=3>

"Fibromyalgia-Symptoms." Web MD. Updated 10 Nov 2005. 10 July 2007 <www.webmd.com/fibromyalgia/tc/Fibromyalgia-Symptoms>.

Fink, G., et. al. "Estrogen control of central neurotransmission: Effect on mood, mental state, and memory." *Cell Molecular Biology* 16 (1996): 325–344.

"Fruit and Vegetables: Do You Get Enough." American Cancer Society. 5 Oct 2007.

<www.cancer.org/docroot/subsite/greatamericans/content/ Fruits_and_Vegetables_Do_You_Get_Enough.asp>.

"Fibromyalgia-Medications." Web MD. Updated 30 Oct 2007. 12 Sept 2008. <www.webmd.com/fibromyalgia/ tc/Fibromyalgia-Medications>.

Gershon, Michael, MD, *The Second Brain,* Harper Perennial, 1998.

Gilliland, Regina, MD "Fibromyalgia." E Medicine. Updated 22 Jan 2007. 29 Aug 2007. <http://www.emedicine. com/pmr/topic47.htm>

Gonzales, G.F., & Carillo, C. "Blood serotonin levels in post-menopausal women: Effects of age and estradiol levels." *Maturitas.* 17. (1993) 23–39.

Hallowell, Edward, MD, and John Ratey, MD *Driven to Distraction.* New York, NY: Touchstone Books, 1994. 274.

Holman, Andrew J. and Robin R. Myers. "A randomized, double-blind, placebo-controlled trial of Pramipexole, a Dopamine Agonist, in patients with fibromyalgia receiving concomitant medications." *Arthritis & Rheumatism* 52:8 (Aug 2005) 2495.

"Inositol." *Inositol.Net.* 18 Aug 2007. <www.inositol.net/inositol.asp>.

Khorram O. et. al. "Activation of immune function by dehydroepiandrosterone (DHEA) in age-advanced men." *J Gerontol A Biol Sci Med Sci.* 52 (1997): M1–7.

Krause, K., Krause et. al. "Fibromyalgia syndrome and attention deficit hyperactivity disorder: Is there a comorbidity and are there consequences for the therapy of fibromyalgia syndrome?" *Journal of Musculoskeletal Pain.* 6:4 (1998) 111–116.

Lang, Janet. *Functional Endocrinology: Balancing Female Hormones Part 1 and 2*. Seminar: May 2006, Atlanta, GA.

Lang, Janet. *Functional Endocrinology: Thyroid, Adrenals, Pancreas, and Male Hormones*. 2006.

Laumann, E, et al, 1999. Sexual Dysfunction in the United States: Prevalence and Predictors. *Journal of the American Medical Association* 281:537–544.

Lee, John. *What Your Doctor May Not Tell You About Menopause*. New York, NY: Warner Books, 1996.

Levine J. "Controlled Trials of Inositol in Psychiatry." *Eur Neuropsychopharmacol*, 7 May 1997. 2:147–155.

Medical University of South Carolina, "Digestive Organs." Updated 7 Feb 2007. 1 Sept 2007. 1. <http://www.ddc.musc.edu/ddc_pub/digestiveOrgans /smallBowel.htm>.

Murray, M. and J. Pizzorno. *Encyclopedia of Natural Medicine*. New York, NY: Prima Health, 1998. 462.

Nadeau, Kathleen, Ph. D. and Patricia Quinn, MD *Understanding Women with AD/HD*. Silver Springs, MD: Advantage Books, 2002.

"Norepinephrine." 29 Aug. 2007. http://dwp.bigplanet.com/nutritionpsych/norepinephrine

Northrup, Christiane. *The Wisdom of Menopause*, New York, NY: Bantam Dell, 2003.

"Omega 3 Fatty Acids." *The George Mateljan Foundation*. 2 Oct 2007. <www.whfoods.com/genpage.php?tname=nutrient&dbid=84>.

"Pain and Depression: Are They Linked?" Mayo Clinic. Updated Oct 2006. 29 Aug 2007

http://www.mayoclinic.com/health/pain-and-depression/AN01449.

Prohealth, Inc. 2 Feb 2009 <http://www.prohealth.com/fibromyalgia/index.cfm?b1=FMWEBO

Puttini, P.S. and I. Caruso. "Primary fibromyalgia syndrome and 5 hydroxy-L-tyrptophan: a 90-day open study." *J Int Med Res.* 20 (1992) 182–189.

Randolph, C.W. *From Hormone Hell to Hormone Well.* Jacksonville Beach, FL: The National Hormone Institute of America, Inc., 2004.

Reiss, Uzzi. *Balancing Natural Hormones.* New York, NY: Pocket Books, 2001.

"Remove, Replace, Reinoculate, Repair: The 4 R Gastrointestinal Support Program." *HealthComm International, Inc.* 1998,< www.healthcomm.com>

Rodriguez, M.M., and G. T. Grossberg. "Estrogen as a psychotherapeutic agent."*Clinical Geriatric Medicine,* 14 (1998): 177–189.

Shames, Richard, Shames, Karlee. *Thyroid Power: Ten Steps to Total Health,* New York, NY: Collins Wellness, 2005.

Shomon, Mary. *The Thyroid Hormone Breakthrough.* New York, NY: Harper Collins, 2006.

"*Stimulant AD/HD Medications.*" National Institute on Drug Abuse. Revised June 2008, Sept 2008. 1 http://www.drugabuse.gov/infofacts/AD/HD.html

"Symptoms of AD/HD." Centers for Disease Control and Prevention. Updated Sept 2005. 17 Sept 2008 < www.cdc.gov/ncbddd/adhd/symptom.htm>

Tavoni A. et. al. "Evaluation of S-adenosylmethionine in primary fibromyalgia. A

double- blind crossover study." *Am J Med.* 83:5A (1987) 107–110.

Taylor, Eldred and Ava Taylor. *Are Your Hormones Making You Sick?* Physician's Natural Medicine, Inc., 2000.

Teitelbaum J. *From Fatigued to Fantastic.* New York, NY: Avery Publishing, 2001.

Van Hartesveldt, C., and J. N. Joyce. "Effects of estrogen on the basil ganglia." N*euroscience and Biobehavioral Reviews.* 10 (1986): 1–14.

Vliet, Elizabeth, MD *Screaming to be Heard.* New York, NY: M. Evans and Company, Inc., 1995.

Watson, Brenda, N.D, C.T, *Renew Your Life.* Renew Life Press and Information Services, 2002.

Watson, Brenda, ND, Smith, Leonard, MD *Gut Solutions.* Renew Life Press and Information Services, 2003.

"Whole Grains: Hearty Options for a Healthy Diet." *Mayo Clinic.* Updated 8 Feb 2008, 5 Oct 2007. . <www.mayoclinic.com/health/whole-grains/NU00204 >.

Wilson, James. *Adrenal Fatigue: The 21st Century Stress Syndrome.* Smart Publications, 2001. 4

Wood, P. "Stress and dopamine: implications for pathophysiology of chronic widespread pain." Medical Hypotheses 62, (2004) 422.

Wood, P. "A reconsideration of the relevance of systemic low-dose ketamine to the pathophysiology of fibromyalgia." *The Journal of Pain.* 7: 9 (2006) 613.

Yen S.S. et. al. "Replacement of DHEA in aging men and women." *Ann NY Acad Sci.* 774 (1995): 128–142.

Yokogoshi H. et. al. "Effect of theanine, r-glutamylethylamide on brain monoamines and striatal dopamine release in conscious rats." *Neurochem Res.* 23 (1998) 667–673.

Contact Information

My Web site address is www.reversingchronicdisease. com. If you are helped from the information in this book, please write and share with me. Also, watch for updated information.

EndNotes

1.   National Fibromyalgia Research Association. 6 Mar 2007. 1 <www.nfra.net/fibromyalgia_definition.php>

2.   "About Fibromyalgia," UCLA Center for Neurovisceral Sciences and Women's Health. 2 July 2008. 1 <www.cns.med.ucla.edu/PatientFibro.htm>

3.   "Fibromyalgia Causes." Mayo Clinic. 4 Oct 2006. 200:1–2. 26 Feb 2007. 1 <www.mayoclinic.com/health/fibromyalgia/DS00079/DSECTION=3>

4.   "Fibromyalgia-Symptoms." Web MD. 10 Nov 2005. 10 July 2007. 1 <www.webmd.com/fibro-myalgia/tc/Fibromyalgia-Symptoms>

5.   "Fibromyalgia Causes." Mayo Clinic. 4 Oct 2006:1–2. 24 Feb 2007. 1 <www.mayoclinic.com/print/fibromyalgia/DS00079/DSECTION=3>,

6.   "Fibromyalgia-Cause." Web MD. 10 Nov 2005. 24 Feb 2007. <www.webmd.com/fibromyal-gia/tc/Fibromyalgia-Topic-Overview>.

7.   Vliet, Elizabeth, MD *Screaming to be Heard*. New York, NY: M. Evans and Company, Inc., 1995. 229.

8.   Vliet. 230.

9.   Teitelbaum, Jacob, MD *From Fatigued To Fantastic*.
     New York, NY: Avery Publishing, 2001. 98–100.

10. Teitelbaum 48.

11. Teitelbaum. 52.

12. "Fibromyalgia-Medications." *Web MD*. 10 July 2009.
     *www.webmd.com/fibromyalgia/guide/fibromyalgia-
     treatment-medications-that-can-and-cant-help*

13. "Fibromyalgia-Medications." *Web MD*. 10 July 2009.
     *www.webmd.com/fibromyalgia/guide/fibromyalgia-
     treatment-medications-that-can-and-cant-help*

14. Teitelbaum 160–168.

15. Teitelbaum 153.

16. Lang, Janet. *Functional Endocrinology:
     Balancing Female Hormone Part 2*,
     Seminar May 2006, Atlanta, GA.

17. Reiss, Uzzi. *Balancing Natural Hormones*.
     New York, N.Y. Pocket Books, 2001, 7.

18. Randolph, C.W. *From Hormone Hell to Hormone
     Well*. Jacksonville Beach, FL: The National
     Hormone Institute of America, Inc., 2004. 57.

19. Randolph 79–80.

20. Lang, Janet. *Functional Endocrinology:
     Balancing Female Hormones Part 1*. 2006. 24.

21. Northrup, Christiane. *The Wisdom of Menopause*,
     New York, N.Y., Bantam Dell, 2003. 279.

22. Lang 28.

23. Randolph 112–113.

24. Randolph 31.

25. Lang 56.

26. Randolph 9.

27. Randolph 32.

28. Dr. Janet Lang Seminar. *Functional Endocrinology: Part 2*, Atlanta, GA. May 2006.

29. Lang 30.

30. Randolph 236–238.

31. Randolph 236.

32. Lang, Janet. *Functional Endocrinology: Thyroid, Adrenals, Pancreas, and Male Hormones.* 2006. III.

33. Archer, J.S. "Estrogen and mood changes via CNS activity," *Menopausal Medicine.* 7 (1999): 4–8.

34. Fink, G., et. al. "Estrogen control of central neurotransmission: Effect on mood, mental state, and memory." *Cell Molecular Biology* 16 (1996): 325–344.

35. Van Hartesveldt, C., and J. N. Joyce. "Effects of estrogen on the basil ganglia." *Neuroscience and Biobehavioral Reviews.* 10 (1986): 1–14.

36. Rodriguez, M.M., and G. T. Grossberg. "Estrogen as a psychotherapeutic agent. ." *Clinical Geriatric Medicine.* 14 (1998): 177–189.

37. Fink, G., Rosie, R., Grace O., Quinn, JP. "Estrogen control of central neurotransmission: Effect on mood, mental state, and memory." *Cell Molecular Biology.* 16 (1996): 325–344.

38. Nadeau, K., Quinn, P. *Understanding Women with AD/HD.* Silver Spring, MD Advantage Books, 2002. p. 89.

39. Gonzales, G.F., & Carillo, C. "Blood serotonin levels in postmenopausal women: Effects of age and estradiol levels." *Maturitas.* 17. (1993) 23–39.

40. Arpels, J.C. "The female brain hypoestrogenic continuum from the premenstrual syndrome to menopause: A hypothesis and review." *Journal of Reproductive Medicine.* 41 (1996): 633–639.

41. Wilson, James. *Adrenal Fatigue: The 21st Century Stress Syndrome.* Smart Publications, 2001. 4.

42. Wilson xxi.

43. Teitelbaum J. *From Fatigued to Fantastic.* New York, N.Y: Avery Publishing, 2001. 31.

44. Lang 15.

45. Wilson 3–4.

46. Lang, Janet. *Functional Endocrinology: Thyroid, Adrenals, Pancreas, and Male Hormones.* 2006. 16.

47. Wilson 27–44.

48. Lang 15–16.

49. Nadeau, Kathleen, Quinn, Patricia. *Understanding Women with AD/HD.* Silver Spring, MD: Advantage Books. 2002. p. 202.

50. Khorram O. et. al. "Activation of immune function by dehydroepiandrosterone (DHEA) in age-advanced men." *J Gerontol A Biol Sci Med Sci.* 52 (1997): M1–7.

51. Yen S.S. et. al. "Replacement of DHEA in aging men and women." *Ann NY Acad Sci.* 774 (1995): 128–142.

52. Lang. 27c.

53. Randolph, C.W. *From Hormone Hell to Hormone Well.* Jacksonville Beach, FL: The National Hormone; Institute of America, Inc. 2004. 26.

54. "Addison's Disease." National Endocrine and Metabolic Diseases Information Services, a service of The National Institute of Diabetes, Digestive and

Kidney Diseases. 13 July 2008. <http://www.endo-crine.niddk.nih.gov/pubs/addison/addison.htm.>

55. Lang 27a b -27c.

56. Shames, Richard, and Karlee Shames. *Thyroid Power: Ten Steps to Total Health*, New York, NY: Collins Wellness, 2005. 108.

57. Shames 288.

58. Shames 16–17.

59. Lee, John. *What Your Doctor May Not Tell You About Menopause*. New York, NY: Warner Books, 1996. 98.

60. Lee 146.

61. Shomon, Mary. *The Thyroid Hormone Breakthrough*. New York, NY: Harper Collins, 2006. 32.

62. Shames 16.

63. Shames 22.

64. Shames 90–92.

65. Randolph, C.W. *From Hormone Hell to Hormone Well*. Jacksonville Beach, FL: The National Hormone; Institute of America, Inc. 2004. 97–98.

66. Randolph 274.

67. Dr. Janet Lang Seminar. *Functional Endocrinology: Part 2*. Atlanta, GA. May 2006.

68. Taylor, Eldred, and Ava Taylor. *Are Your Hormones Making You Sick?*, Physician's Natural Medicine, Inc., 2000. 52–53.

69. Company Biography. 27 Jan. 2008 <www.diagnostechs.com/main/htm>

70. Laumann, E, et al, 1999. "Sexual Dysfunction in the United States: Prevalence and Predictors." *Journal of the American Medical Association*. 281:537–544.

71. Dr. Janet Lang Seminar. *Functional Endocrinology: Part 2*, Atlanta, GA. May 2006.

72. Dr. Janet Lang Seminar. *Functional Endocrinology: Part 2*, Atlanta, GA. May 2006.

73. "Symptoms of AD/HD." Centers for Disease Control and Prevention. Updated Sept 2005. 17 Sept 2008. 1–2. <www.cdc.gov/ncbddd/adhd/symptom.htm >

74. "Diagnosis of AD/HD in Adults." National Resource Center on AD/HD. Sept 2005, cited 17 Sept 2008. 1–2< http://www.help4adhd.org/en/treatment>

75. Nadeau, Kathleen, Ph. D. and Patricia Quinn, MD *Understanding Women with AD/HD*. Silver Springs, MD.: Advantage Books 2002, 4.

76.   Hallowell, Edward, MD, and John Ratey, MD *Driven to Distraction*. New York, NY: Touchstone Books, 1994. 274.

77. Nadeau 202

78. Amen, Daniel, MD *Healing ADD*. New York, N.Y.: G.P. Putman's Sons, 2001. 261–262.

79. "Diagnosis of AD/HD in Adults." National Resource Center on AD/HD. 09/07/08. 1 http://www.help4adhd.org/en/treatment/guides/WWK9 [Jenn, I added remaining reference.]

80. "*Stimulant AD/HD Medications*." National Institute on Drug Abuse. Revised June 2008, Sept 2008. 1 <http://www.drugabuse.gov/infofacts/AD/HD.html>

81. Nadeau 191

82. Nadeau 218

83. Nadeau 88

84. Yaffe, K., Sawaya, G., Lieberburg, I., Grady, D., "Estrogen therapy in postmenopausal women: Effects

on cognitive function and demential. *Journal of the American Medical Association.* 279 (1998) 688–695.

85. Nadeau 97

86. Murphy, D. DeCarli, C., McIntosh, A. "Sex differences in brain morphology and metabolism: An in-vivo quantitative magnetic reasonance imaging and positron emission tomography study on the effects of aging." *Archives of Geriatric Psychiatry* 53 (1996) 585–594.

87. Nadeau 94–95

88. Nadeau 55

89. Amen, Daniel, MD "The Brain Place." The Amen Clinic. 27 Sept 2008. http://amenclinics.com/bp/articles.php?articleID=10

90. Vliet, Elizabeth. *Screaming to be Heard.* New York, NY: M. Evans Co., 2000. 68.

91. Wood, P. "Stress and dopamine: implications for pathophysiology of chronic widespread pain." Medical Hypotheses 62, (2004) 422.

92. Wood, P. "A reconsideration of the relevance of systemic low-dose ketamine to the pathophysiology of fibromyalgia." *The Journal of Pain.* 7: 9 (2006) 613.

93. Wood. "A reconsideration of the relevance of systemic low-dose ketamine to the pathophysiology of fibromyalgia." 611.

94. Holman, Andrew J. and Robin R. Myers. "A randomized, double-blind, placebo-controlled trial of Pramipexole, a Dopamine Agonist, in patients with fibromyalgia receiving concomitant medications." *Arthritis & Rheumatism* 52:8 (August 2005) 2495.

95. Vliet 230.

96.   Devonshire, R and J. Kelly. "Pioneer Treatments
       for Fibromyalgia and Chronic Fatique Syndrome."
       HealthWatch Treatment Guide. Sept 2003. 16
       Aug 2007. <www.immunesupport.com.>

97.   Krause, K., Krause et. al. "Fibromyalgia syndrome
       and attention deficit hyperactivity disorder: Is
       there a comorbidity and are there consequences
       for the therapy of fibromyalgia syndrome?" *Journal
       of Musculoskeletal Pain.* 6:4 (1998) 111–116.

98.   Teitelbaum, J. *From Fatigued to Fantastic.*
       New York: Avery Publishing, 2001. 153.

99.   Tavoni A. et. al. "Evaluation of
       S-adenosylmethionine in primary fibro-
       myalgia. A double- blind crossover study."
       Am J Med. 83:5A (1987) 107–110.

100.   *Alternative Medicine Review*, 3:3 (1998) 224.

101.   Puttini, P.S. and I. Caruso. "Primary fibromyalgia
       syndrome and 5 hydroxy-L-tyrptophan: a 90-day
       open study." *J Int Med Res.* 20 (1992) 182–189.

102.   Caruso I. et. al. "Double-blind study of
       5-Hydroxytryptophan versus placebo in treat-
       ment of primary fibromyalgia syndrome."
       J Int Med Res. 18 (1990) 201–209.

103.   Yokogoshi H. et. al. "Effect of theanine,
       r-glutamylethylamide on brain monoam-
       ines and striatal dopamine release in conscious
       rats." *Neurochem Res.* 23 (1998) 667–673.

104.   Murray, M. and J. Pizzorno. *Encyclopedia of Natural
       Medicine.* New York: Prima Health, 1998. 462.

105.   "Pain and Depression: Are They Linked?" Mayo
       Clinic. Oct 2006. 29 Aug 2007. <http://www.may-
       oclinic.com/health/pain-and-depression/AN01449.>

106. Gilliland, Regina, MD "Fibromyalgia." E
     Medicine. Updated 22 Jan 2007. 29 Aug 2007
     <http://www.emedicine.com/pmr/topic47.htm>

107. "Inositol." Inositol.Net. 18 Aug 2007
     <www.inositol.net/inositol.asp>.

108. "Inositol." Inositol.Net. 18 Aug 2007
     <www.inositol.net/inositol.asp>.

109. Levine J. "Controlled Trials of Inositol in Psychiatry."
     Eur Neuropsychopharmacol. 1997 May 7. (2):147–155.

110. Gershon, Michael, MD, *The Second Brain*,
     New York, NY: Harper Perennial, 1998. 70.

111. Medical University of South Carolina,
     "Digestive Organs." Updated 7 Feb 2007.
     1 Sept 2007 1.<http://www.ddc.musc.edu/
     ddc_pub/digestiveOrgans /smallBowel.htm>

112. Ibid. 1.

113. Watson, Brenda, N.D, C.T. *Renew Your Life*. Renew
     Life Press and Information Services, 2002. 3.

114. "Remove, Replace, Reinoculate, Repair: The 4 R
     Gastrointestinal Support Program." HealthComm
     International, Inc. 1998. 1–6 <www.healthcomm.
     com>

115. Braly, James, MD "IgG ELISA Delayed Food Allergy
     Testing." 3 Sept 2007 <http://www.drbralyallergyre-
     lief.com/igg.html>

116. Watson, Brenda, ND Smith, Leonard, MD *Gut
     Solutions*. Renew Life Press and Information Services,
     2003. 219.

117. Watson. *Gut Solutions*. 4–5.

118. "Fruit and Vegetables: Do You Get Enough."
     American Cancer Society. 5 Oct 2007.
     <www.cancer.org/docroot/subsite/greatameri-

cans/content/Fruits_and_Vegetables_
Do_You_Get_Enough.asp>.

119. "Whole Grains: Hearty Options for a Healthy Diet."
Mayo Clinic. Updated 8 Feb 2008, 5 Oct 2007. <www.
mayoclinic.com/health/whole-grains/NU00204 >

120. "Omega 3 Fatty Acids." The George
Mateljan Foundation. 2 Oct. 2007. 2
Oct. 2007. <www.whfoods.com/gen-
page.php?tname=nutrient&dbid=84>